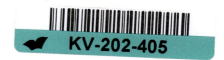
The Kidney and Hypertension in Pregnancy

For Churchill Livingstone

Publisher Mike Parkinson
Project Editor Dilys Jones
Copy Editor Prunella Theaker
Production Controller Debra Barrie
Sales Promotion Executive Kathy Crawford

The Kidney and Hypertension in Pregnancy

Priscilla S. Kincaid-Smith DSC MD FRCP FRACP FRCPA
Professor of Medicine, University of Melbourne; Director of
Nephrology, Royal Melbourne Hospital; Honorary Consulting
Physician, Royal Women's Hospital, Melbourne, Australia

Kenneth F. Fairley MD FRCP FRACP
Professorial Associate in Medicine, University of Melbourne
and Department of Medicine, Royal Melbourne Hospital;
Physician, Royal Women's Hospital, Melbourne, Australia

CHURCHILL LIVINGSTONE
EDINBURGH LONDON MADRID MELBOURNE NEW YORK AND TOKYO 1993

CHURCHILL LIVINGSTONE
Medical Division of Longman Group UK Limited

Distributed in the United States of America by Churchill
Livingstone Inc., 650 Avenue of the Americas, New York,
N.Y. 10011, and by associated companies, branches and
representatives throughout the world.

First published 1993

ISBN 0-443-04536-4

British Library Cataloguing in Publication Data
A catalogue record for this book is available from the British
Library.

Library of Congress Cataloging in Publication Data
Kincaid-Smith, Priscilla, 1926–
    The kidney and hypertension in pregnancy/Priscilla S.
Kincaid–Smith, Kenneth F. Fairley.
        p.   cm.
    Includes index.
    ISBN 0-443-04536-4
    1. Kidney diseases in pregnancy. 2. Hypertension in
pregnancy. I. Fairley, Kenneth F. II. Title.
    [DNLM: 1. Hypertension—in pregnancy. 2. Kidney—
physiology. 3. Kidney Diseases—in pregnancy. 4.
Pregnancy Complications. WQ 240 K51k]
    RG580.K5K55   1993
    616.6'1—dc20
    DNLM/DLC
    for Library of Congress   92-49139

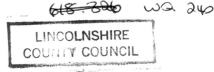
The
publisher's
policy is to use
**paper manufactured
from sustainable forests**

Produced by Longman Singapore Publishers (Pte) Ltd.
Printed in Singapore

Contents

1. Historical

The association between dropsy and kidney disease ('durities in renibus') was described by William de Saliceto in the thirteenth century; however, proteinuria was first noted some 500 years later when Bright in his outstanding contribution documented in detail the potentially ominous significance of proteinuria in what became known as Bright's disease. Proteinuria in association with preeclampsia was first described by Rayer (1841). In 1843 Simpson in Edinburgh and Lever at Guy's Hospital (Lever 1843, Simpson 1843) both described proteinuria in eclampsia/preeclampsia. Lever described proteinuria in 9 of 10 women with eclampsia and also made important observations about its rapid abatement after delivery (Lever 1843).

Matters relating to pregnancy and delivery featured very little in medical texts until the invention of the obstetric forceps. Although forceps were in use in the seventeenth century their use was vehemently attacked particularly by midwives. Early obstetricians were dubbed 'man midwives' and were most unwelcome in the labour room. Early in the eighteenth century William Smellie set up a school of midwifery for doctors in London and thereafter, at least in the United Kingdom, medical practitioners (and hence men) gradually assumed control of complicated deliveries.

One of the best accounts of the history of eclampsia is that of Chesley (1976). Chesley delves into the recognition of eclampsia in the ancient Egyptian, Chinese, Indian and Greek Literature and quotes Mahomed's report on sphygmographic tracings in which he wrongly concluded that hypertension was a feature found in all pregnant women (Mahomed 1874). Ballantyne, a decade later, also on the basis of sphygmographic tracings, concluded that the arterial blood pressure was considerably elevated in 1 preeclamptic and 2 eclamptic women (Ballantyne 1885). Towards the end of the century more accurate blood pressure measurements became available; Cook & Briggs (1903) observed that the blood pressure was little altered in normal pregnancy and made the important observation that proteinuria when it occurred was usually associated with hypertension.

Oedema — the other sign of preeclampsia and eclampsia — received little attention in the literature but could not have escaped notice because it is usually so severe (Chesley 1976).

Any clear-cut separation of eclampsia and preeclampsia from chronic hypertension and renal disease was delayed until well into the twentieth century. Lever, as early as 1843, noted that the proteinuria of eclampsia disappeared while that of Bright's disease persisted after pregnancy, but in spite of this astute early observation confusion persisted for almost a century about so-called 'nephritic toxaemia'.

Herrick (1932) recognized hypertension as both a frequent and important occurrence in the so-called 'toxaemias of pregnancies' and was one of the first to question the use of the word 'toxaemia'. He thought that many cases of essential hypertension in pregnancy had been erroneously called chronic nephritis which he thought accounted for only a small number of cases (Herrick & Tillman 1936).

Dieckmann (1952) also commented on the rarity of renal disease in patients with preeclampsia, stating that not more than 2% of cases have underlying renal disease. More recent studies based on renal biopsy findings suggest that the figure may be much higher, some 22% of biopsies showing evidence of underlying renal disease (Fisher et al 1981).

One important aspect of the diagnosis of pre-eclampsia is the recognition that the blood pressure falls in normal pregnancy. This was first documented by Hare & Karn (1929). This observation led to a definition of an abnormal blood pressure based in part on a rise observed during pregnancy in the individual patient.

Browne & Dodds (1942) noted that if the blood pressure rose above 130/70 before 20 weeks gestation preeclampsia occurred in 18% of cases, and if the blood pressure was recorded above 150/100 before 20 weeks 32% of women developed preeclampsia.

REFERENCES

Ballantyne J W 1885 Sphygmographic tracings in puerperal eclampsia. Edinburgh Medical Journal 30 (2): 1007–1021.

Browne F J, Dodds G H 1942 Pregnancy in the patient with chronic hypertension. Journal of Obstetrics and Gynaecology of the British Empire 49: 1–17.

Chesley L 1976 Historical developments. In: Freedman E A (ed) Blood pressure, oedema and proteinuria in pregnancy. Alan R, Liss, New York, p 19–66

Cook H W, Briggs J B 1903 Clinical observations on blood pressure. Johns Hopkins Hospital Report 11: 451–531.

Dieckmann W J 1952 Toxaemias of pregnancy, 2nd edn. CV Mosby, St Louis.

Fisher K A, Luger A, Spargo BH et al 1981 Hypertension in pregnancy: clinico–pathological correlations and remote prognosis. Medicine 60: 267–276.

Hare D C, Karn N 1929 An investigation of blood-pressure, pulse-rate and the response to exercise during normal pregnancy, and some observations after confinement. Quarterly Journal of Medicine 22: 381–404

Herrick W W 1932 The toxaemias of pregnancy and their end results from the viewpoint of internal medicine. Illinois Medical Journal 62: 210

Herrick W W, Tillman A J B 1936 The mild toxaemias of late pregnancy: their relation to cardiovascular and renal disease. American Journal of Obstetrics and Gynecology 31: 832

Lever J C W 1843 Case of puerperal convulsions, with remarks. Guy's Hospital Reports 1 (second series): 459

Mahomed F A 1874 The aetiology of Bright's disease and the prealbuminuric stage. British Medical Journal 1: 585–586

Rayer P 1841 Traite des maladies des reins et des alterations de la secretion urinaire. J B Baillière, Paris, vol II: 399–407

Simpson J Y 1843 Contributions to the pathology and treatment of the uterus. London and Edinburgh Monthly Journal of Medical Science 3: 1009–1027

2. Anatomical and morphological changes in the kidney in pregnancy

2.1 INCREASE IN RENAL SIZE

Evidence that the kidney increases in size during pregnancy is largely dependent upon imaging studies done in the early postpartum period. Both Bailey & Rolleston (1971) and Kauppila et al (1972) observed that the kidney in the puerperium was larger than the normal values recorded in non-pregnant women (Hodson 1972). Bailey & Rolleston (1971) repeated intravenous pyelograms 6 months after delivery in a small number of women and found a mean shrinkage of 0.8 cm in renal length compared with the studies in the puerperium.

It is not yet altogether clear which structures within the kidney enlarge during pregnancy and to what extent an increase in renal vascular volume (associated with increased blood flow) and an increase in interstitial fluid contribute to the increase in renal size. There is no obvious increase in interstitial tissue seen on renal biopsies in pregnant women. Sheehan made careful measurements on kidneys obtained at autopsy from women dying during pregnancy or in the early postpartum period. Glomerular diameter in his control or 'non-toxaemic' group was 195 µm; however, he pointed to the difficulties in assessing if this was large because of the wide range of measurements in previous studies in non-pregnant women, perhaps due to methods of processing material for histological examination (Sheehan & Lynch 1973).

In the rat and the mouse renal weight is increased during pregnancy. Part of this change is due to hypertrophy of cells, but it has been suggested it may partly be related to an increase in renal water content (Mathews 1977, Davison & Lindheimer 1980).

2.2 DILATATION OF THE CALYCES, PELVIS AND URETER

The most striking anatomical change which occurs in the kidney during pregnancy is the dilatation of the renal calyces and pelvis and the ureters (Fig. 2.2–1). First recognition of this dilatation is attributed to Cruveilhier (1841). It was first documented radiographically in 1925 (Kretschmer & Heaney 1925). This change is more common and more pronounced on the right side and is present in 90% of pregnant women (Crabtree 1952, Fainstat 1963, Bailey & Rolleston 1971,

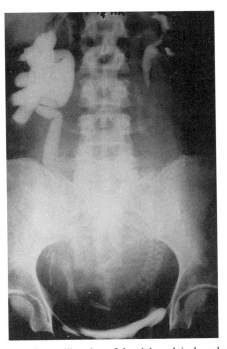

Fig. 2.2–1 Gross dilatation of the right pelvicalyceal system and ureter in pregnancy.

Kauppila et al 1972, Fayad et al 1973, Lindheimer & Katz 1977, Roberts 1978, Fried 1979).

The early observations were based on radiographic findings, but ultrasound now allows more extensive studies and is of particular value in serial observations. Nuclear scans using radioisotopes have shown an 'obstructive' pattern in the dilated urinary tract during pregnancy (Baird et al 1966, Laakso 1967). A comparison of findings on an intravenous pyelogram and those on a renogram found that renography was more sensitive (Fayad et al 1973); however, ultrasound would now be the method of choice for documenting the degree of dilatation because it avoids the use of radiation and radioisotopes.

Obstruction has probably been favoured over a hormonal cause as the underlying mechanism of the dilated urinary tract in pregnancy because the dilatation is accompanied by hypertrophy of muscle and an increase in connective tissue and by a decrease in peristalsis. The changes may, however, be seen in the first trimester which favours an hormonal mechanism contributing to the dilatation.

Changes in smooth muscle occur in other organs in pregnancy which also implies an hormonal mechanism. The role of relaxin in ureteric dilatation has not been studied but this is one of the hormones produced in pregnancy which could play a role in dilatation of the renal tract. The most powerful argument that ureteric dilatation in pregnancy is due to hormonal factors rather than obstruction is the demonstration by Van Wagenen & Jenkins (1939) that in primates, after removal of the fetus, the ureter dilatation increases in the presence of an intact placenta.

Dure-Smith (1970) favours a major role for obstruction in the dilatation of the urinary tract seen in pregnancy. He demonstrated that the dilatation is above the point where the ureter crosses the iliac artery at the pelvic brim, and he demonstrated a filling defect in the ureter at this site.

The dilatation of the urinary tract leads to some degree of stasis and to increase in dead space. It has been suggested that this may predispose to infection. Perhaps the strongest evidence that this may be so is that of Fairley et al (1966), who demonstrated that, in bacteriuric women with unilateral dilatation of ureter pelvis and calyces, the infection was always localized to the side of the dilatation.

Lindheimer & Katz (1977) have pointed out that the dead space created by the dilatation may interfere with renal function tests.

Dilatation of the ureter calyces and pelvis may persist for 3 months after pregnancy (Crabtree 1952); persistent dilatation beyond that time is observed in a proportion of women and is not necessarily associated with either bacteriuria or symptomatic infection (Spiro 1970).

REFERENCES

Bailey R R, Rolleston G L 1971 Kidney length and ureteric dilatation in the puerperium. Journal of Obstetrics and Gynaecology of the British Commonwealth 78: 55–61
Baird D T, Gasson P W, Doig A 1966 The renogram in pregnancy. American Journal of Obstetrics and Gynecology 95: 597–603
Crabtree F 1952 Urological diseases of pregnancy. Williams & Williams, Baltimore
Cruveilhier J 1841 Descriptive anatomy. Whitaker, London
Davison J M, Lindheimer M D 1980 Changes in renal haemodynamics and kidney weight during pregnancy in the unanaesthetized rat. Journal of Physiology 301: 129–136
Dure-Smith P 1970 Pregnancy dilatation of the urinary tract. Radiology 96: 545–550
Fainstat T 1963 Ureteral dilatation in pregnancy: a review. Obstetrical; and Gynecological Survey 18: 845–860
Fairley K F, Bond A G, Adey F D et al 1966 The site of infection in pregnancy bacteriuria. Lancet 1: 939–941.
Fayad M M, Upissef A F, Zahran M et al 1973 The ureterocalyceal system in normal pregnancy. Acta Obstetricia et Gynecologica Scandinavica 52: 69–76
Fried A M 1979 Hydronephrosis of pregnancy: ultrasonographic study and classification of asymptomatic women. American Journal of Obstetrics and Gynecology 135: 1066–1070
Hodson C J 1972 Radiology of the kidney. In: D. Black (ed) Renal disease, 3rd edn. Blackwell Scientific, Oxford, ch 8, p 213–249
Kauppila A, Satuli R, Vuorinen P 1972 Ureteric dilatation and renal cortical index after normal and preeclamptic pregnancies. Acta Obstetricia and Gynecologica Scandinavica 51: 147–153
Kretschmer H L, Heaney N S 1925 Dilatation of the ureter and kidney pelvis during pregnancy. Journal of the American Medical Association 85:406
Laakso L 1967 Isotope renography on parturients. Acta Obstetricia and Gynecologica Scandinavica 46 (suppl 5): 5–104
Lindheimer M D, Katz A I 1977 Kidney function and disease in pregnancy. Lea & Febiger, Philadelphia, p 7
Mathews B F 1977 Growth of the maternal kidneys in pregnant mice. Journal of Physiology 273: 84P

Roberts J A 1978 Hydronephrosis of pregnancy. Urology 8: 1–4

Sheehan H L, Lynch J B (eds) 1973 Pathology of toxaemia of pregnancy. Churchill Livingstone, Edinburgh, p 47

Spiro F I 1970 Ureteric dilatation in nonpregnant women. Proceedings of the Royal Society of Medicine 63: 462

Van Wagenen G, Jenkins R H 1939 An experimental examination of factors causing ureteral dilatation of pregnancy. Journal of Urology 42: 1010–1021

3. Physiological adaptation in the kidney in pregnancy

3.1 ALTERATIONS IN RENAL HAEMODYNAMICS

The considerable alterations in renal haemo-dynamics which occur during pregnancy to some extent reflect major cardiovascular alterations such as peripheral vasodilatation, a fall in systemic blood pressure and a 30% increase in cardiac output (Walters et al 1966).

Early data concerning increased renal blood flow during pregnancy came from Bucht (1951). He reported substantial increases in renal blood flow and confirmed, using renal vein catheteriz-ation, that renal extraction of para-aminohippurate, the substance which he used to determine renal blood flow, was 98% in pregnancy as in the non-pregnant state. Numerous subsequent studies confirmed Bucht's observations, and although there was some early disagreement about the extent and sequence of the alterations these appear to have been resolved.

Renal blood flow increases by some 80% be-tween conception and the second trimester (Dunlop 1981) (Fig. 3.1–1). Some of the dis-agreement about renal flow changes relates to the posture of the patient during the test. Chesley & Sloan (1964) demonstrated a 20% reduction in effective renal plasma flow (ERPF) in the supine position compared with the left lateral position. More recent studies confirm that posture may affect ERPF (Ezimokhai et al 1981). These same authors also demonstrated a progressive fall in ERPF measured in the left lateral position from week 29 to week 37.

Accompanying the increase in renal blood flow in pregnancy there is a substantial increase in glomerular filtration rate (GFR) (Fig. 3.1–1).

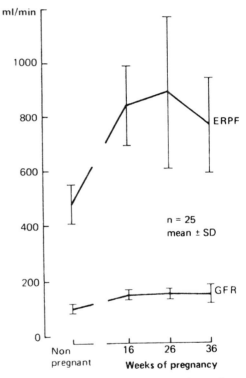

Fig. 3.1–1 Changes in the effective renal plasma flow (ERPF) and glomerular filtration rate (GFR) during pregnancy. (From Dunlop 1981, with permission.)

The creatinine clearance rises by about 50% in the first trimester and remains elevated until the last few weeks of pregnancy. (Sims & Krantz 1958, Ezimokhai et al 1981, Dunlop 1981).

Filtration fraction falls in early pregnancy due to a lesser increase in GFR than in ERPF. It rises again in late pregnancy (Dunlop 1981).

The 24 h creatinine clearance is usually used clinically to determine the GFR. While tubular secretion of creatinine introduces some inaccuracy and the 24 h creatinine clearance gives lower values for the GFR than are obtained using inulin infusion, the convenience of the 24 h creatinine clearance has clearly established it as the method of choice for clinical studies. The creatinine clearance increases by 25% in the first 4 weeks of pregnancy and by 45% by 9 weeks' gestation. The level remains raised until the third trimester when it falls progressively to non-pregnant values (Davison & Dunlop 1980, Davison & Noble 1981).

3.2 PROTEIN EXCRETION IN NORMAL PREGNANCY

An increase in urinary protein excretion is one of the cardinal signs of preeclampsia and hence normal upper limits of urinary protein excretion and albumin excretion in pregnancy have special significance.

Protein excretion is increased in pregnancy above the normal values in non-pregnant women. The upper limit of normal during pregnancy is usually taken to be 300 mg in 24 h, which is about double the upper limit of excretion of protein in non-pregnant women (Davison 1983). Our experience over the past 30 years suggests that an upper limit of 0.3 g/24 h is incorrect for normal pregnant women and that the correct level is close to that of non-pregnant women, namely 0.15 g/24 h. The vast majority of normal pregnant women have levels below 0.15 g/24 h and setting the level at 0.3 g/24 h results in proteinuria as an early sign of preeclampsia being missed in some patients.

Most methods for estimating protein in the urine detect both filtered 'glomerular' proteins and the major tubular protein found in the urine, namely the Tamm Horsfall protein which is secreted by cells in the distal tubule.

Protein in the urine is filtered through the glomerulus by a 'selective process' and then subjected to a non-selective reabsorption process (Pesce & First 1979). About 10 g of filtered protein are reabsorbed so that only about 150 mg of protein normally appear in the urine. Tamm Horsfall protein is a mucoprotein and constitutes 20–30% of the protein found in normal urine.

Normally less than 40 mg of albumin are excreted in 24 h, and the ratio of albumin to creatinine, which avoids the need to do a 24 h urine collection, has been recommended as a method of estimating glomerular permeability (Barrat 1983).

The appearance of preeclampsia is associated with an increase in urinary albumin excretion and a reduction in Tamm Horsfall protein excretion, so that accurate assessment of albumin excretion in pregnancy is desirable although not routinely available in all areas at this time (Lopes-Espinoza et al 1986).

3.3 RENAL TUBULAR FUNCTION

The substantial increase in GFR during pregnancy is inevitably accompanied by an increased filtered load; hence changes in tubular function are necessary to avoid considerable potential loss of various substances which are in the glomerular filtrate.

3.3.1 Sodium excretion

The filtered load of sodium increases from 20 000 to 30 000 mmol/day during pregnancy (Lindheimer & Katz 1977). To avoid massive sodium loss this increased filtered load of sodium requires a considerable increase in sodium reabsorption by the renal tubule in pregnant women.

Many factors influence sodium excretion during pregnancy and, because sodium is the major factor regulating volume homeostasis, these factors are discussed under 3.5.1. Both proximal and distal renal tubular sodium reabsorption is increased during pregnancy (Thomsen & Olesen 1984, Atherton et al 1987).

3.3.2 Glucose excretion

Early workers attributed the increased excretion of glucose in pregnancy to the increase in GFR and hence the increase glucose load delivered to the tubule. It was assumed that the load exceeded the tubular reabsorptive capacity (Welsh & Sims 1960).

Some 5% of filtered glucose is not reabsorbed by the tubule and this leads to glycosuria in some pregnant women. Women with glycosuria in pregnancy have been shown to have a defective absorption of glucose which is reversed after pregnancy (Davison & Hytten 1987).

Hormonal alterations may play a part in pregnancy glycosuria which occurs in spite of normal blood glucose levels.

Although pregnancy glycosuria has been assumed to be a physiological rather than a pathological change, some adverse effects have been documented in association with glycosuria (Chen et al 1976).

3.3.3 Uric acid excretion

Uric acid is filtered by the glomerulus and is both reabsorbed and secreted by the renal tubule. Reabsorption takes place in the proximal and distal tubules.

Pregnant women excrete more uric acid than do non-pregnant women (Dunlop & Davison 1977, Boyle et al 1966); however, they probably do not produce more uric acid (Seitchik et al 1958).

The serum uric acid falls in pregnancy and while the fall in urea and creatinine probably reflect the rise in GFR the low serum uric acid level may reflect a lower tubular reabsorption, hence higher uric acid excretion. Tubular reabsorption of uric acid increases as pregnancy advances and the serum urate concentration may be in the normal non-pregnant range by the third trimester (Dunlop & Davison 1977).

A rise in uric acid above the level anticipated in a normal pregnancy is an important feature of preeclampsia, as discussed below.

3.3.4 Amino acid excretion

Amino acid excretion increases during pregnancy (Hytten & Cheyne 1972) and can reach levels as high as 2 g/day.

Certain amino acids — namely, histidine, glycine, threonine, serine and alanine — are lost in large amounts in the urine in late pregnancy. Up to 50% of the filtered load of histidine and glycine may be excreted in the urine. Page et al (1955) noted that histidine may disappear from the urine during preeclampsia, which adds clinical

significance to the physiological changes in amino acid excretion during pregnancy.

3.3.5 Potassium excretion

Plasma aldosterone levels are elevated in normal pregnancy and it might be assumed that this would cause excessive tubular potassium loss; however, this does not occur.

In the same way that pregnant women appear resistant to the circulating levels of aldosterone, they do not show the usual kaliuresis produced by exogenous administration of mineralocorticoids (Ehrlich & Lindheimer 1972).

Women with diseases associated with potassium loss, such as primary aldosteronism, may show improvement in potassium levels during pregnancy (Biglieri & Slaton 1967).

3.3.6 Acid excretion

The normal blood pH rises during pregnancy to 7.42–7.44, possibly as a result of hyperventilation; arterial PCO_2 also decreases (Lim et al 1976, Fadel et al 1979).

Tubular urinary acidification mechanisms appear to be intact in pregnancy (Assali et al 1955, Lim et al 1976).

3.4 RENAL CONCENTRATING CAPACITY

Although one might anticipate impairment of renal concentrating capacity as a result of the large filtered load of solute in pregnancy, the studies that have compared maximum osmolality after dehydration or desmopressin (DDAVP) show only slight reduction in concentrating capacity in pregnancy. Mean non-pregnant and pregnant values are given in Table 3.4–1.

3.5 WATER EXCRETION AND OSMOREGULATION DURING PREGNANCY

Plasma osmolality falls in the first 10 weeks of pregnancy to a level which is 8–10 mosm/kg below the prepregnancy value for that patient (Davison et al 1981) (Fig. 3.5–1). This relatively low plasma osmolality persists through pregnancy.

Table 3.4–1 Urinary concentrating ability in pregnant women (adapted from Lindheimer & Katz 1985, with permission)

Source	Maximum U_{osm} (mosm/kg)		Comments
	Non-pregnant	Pregnant	
Davison et al (1981)	854 ± 107 (6)	752 ± 110 (6)	Dehydrated 17 h
Hutchon et al (1982)	1141 ± 223 (7)	826 ± 223 (7)	Dehydrated 15 h
	1109 ± 225 (7)	932 ± 169 (27)	Received desmopressin (DDAVP) without dehydration

U_{osm} = urine osmolality

A decrease in osmolality of this degree would normally cause a massive water diuresis due to inhibition of vasopressin secretion; however, this does not occur in pregnancy. The thresholds for vasopressin secretion and thirst decrease by approximately 8–10 mosm/kg, which corresponds to the decrease in osmolality observed during pregnancy (Davison et al 1984). Water excretion during pregnancy is very dependent on posture. Urine flow reduces when the position changes from the left lateral to the supine position (Pritchard et al 1955, Lindheimer 1970).

The mean vasopressin concentration in plasma is increased in normal pregnancy (Weir et al 1976) and the urine of pregnant women contains a vasopressinase thought to be a of placental origin (Rosenbloom et al 1975).

3.5.1 Volume regulation in pregnancy

Total body water increases during pregnancy by 6–8 l, 60–70% of which is extracellular. Sodium is retained during pregnancy with a cumulative gain of sodium of about 950 mEq (Hytten & Leitch 1971). These volume estimations were carried out on non-oedematous women and, as Robertson pointed out some 20 years ago, 80% of pregnant women develop some oedema during gestation (Robertson 1971). The mean plasma volume in pregnancy increases progressively from the first trimester through to term by almost 50% (Fig. 3.5.1–1) (Pirani et al 1973).

The mechanisms controlling intracellular and extracellular volume during pregnancy are poorly understood but renal sodium handling is a major determinant of the changes that occur.

Historically there has been a view that sodium and water retention during pregnancy may play a part in the aetiology of preeclampsia, and both sodium restriction and diuretics were used in an attempt to prevent preeclampsia. In 1958, Robinson challenged this view and recommended salt supplements for preeclampsia; more recently, Lindheimer et al (1977) have suggested that pregnant women may be subtle salt wasters.

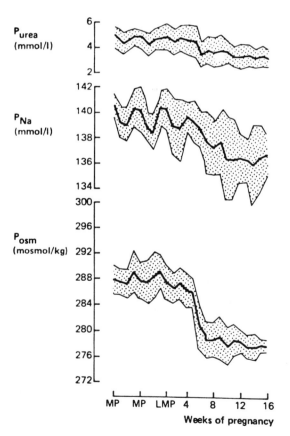

Fig. 3.5–1 Changes in plasma urea, sodium and osmolality in early pregnancy. (From Davison et al 1981, with permission.)

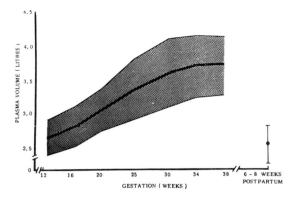

Fig. 3.5.1–1 Changes in plasma volume in pregnancy. (From Pirani et al 1973, with permission.)

Several factors including high oestrogen (Digham 1958) and plasma desoxycorticosterone levels (Nolten et al 1978) may enhance sodium retention during pregnancy. The increase in aldosterone secretion rate during pregnancy provides another potentially potent salt retaining mechanism (Weinberger et al 1976, Nolten et al 1978).

REFERENCES

Assali N S, Herzig D, Singh B P 1955 Renal response to ammonium chloride acidosis in normal and toxaemic pregnancies. Journal of Applied Physiology 7:367–374

Atherton J C, Bobinski H, Davison J M 1987 Renal fluid handling and plasma atrial natriuretic peptide in human pregnancy. Journal of Physiology 387: 90P

Barrat M 1983 Proteinuria. British Medical Journal 287: 1489–1490

Biglieri E G, Slaton Jr P E 1967 Pregnancy and primary aldosteronism. Journal of Clinical Endocrinology and Metabolism 27: 1628

Boyle J A, Campbell S, Duncan A M et al 1966 Serum uric acid levels in normal pregnancy with observations on the renal excretion of urate in pregnancy. Journal of Clinical Pathology 19: 501

Bucht H 1951 Studies on renal function in man with special reference to glomerular filtration and renal plasma flow in pregnancy. Scandinavian Journal of Clinical and Laboratory Investigation 3 (suppl): 1–64

Chen W W, Sese L, Tantakasen P et al 1976 Pregnancy associated with renal glucosuria. Obstetrics and Gynecology 47: 3740

Chesley L C, Sloan D M 1964 The effect of posture on renal function in late pregnancy. American Journal of Obstetrics and Gynecology 89: 754–759

Davison J M 1983 The kidney in pregnancy: a review. Journal of the Royal Society of Medicine 76: 485–501

Davison J M, Dunlop W 1980 Renal haemodynamics and tubular function in normal human pregnancy. Kidney International 18: 152–161

Davison J M, Hytten F E 1987 Can normal pregnancy damage your health? British Journal of Obstetrics and Gynaecology 94: 385–386

Davison J M, Noble M C B 1981 Serial changes in 24 hour creatinine clearance during normal menstrual cycles and the first trimester of pregnancy. British Journal of Obstetrics and Gynaecology 88: 10–17

Davison J M, Vallotton M B, Lindheimer M D 1981 Plasma osmolality and urinary concentration and dilution during and after pregnancy: evidence that lateral recumbency inhibits maximal urinary concentrating ability. British Journal of Obstetrics and Gynaecology 88: 472–479

Davison J M, Gillmore E A, Durr J et al 1984 Altered osmotic thresholds for vasopressin secretion and thirst in human pregnancy. American Journal of Physiology 246: F105–109

Digham W S, Voskian J, Assali N S 1958 Effects of oestrogens on renal haemodynamics and excretion of electrolytes in human subjects. Journal of Clinical Endocrinology and Metabolism 16: 1032–1040

Dunlop W 1981 Serial changes in renal haemodynamics during normal human pregnancy. British Journal of Obstetrics and Gynaecology 88: 1–9

Dunlop W, Davison J M 1977 The effect of normal pregnancy upon the renal handling of uric acid. British Journal of Obstetrics and Gynaecology 84: 13–21

Ehrlich E N, Lindheimer M D 1972 Effect of administered mineralocorticoid on ACTH in pregnant women. Attenuation of the kaliuretic influence on mineralocorticoid during pregnancy. Journal of Clinical Investigation 51: 1301–1309

Ezimokhai M, Davison J M, Phillips P R et al 1981 Non-postural serial changes in renal function during the third trimester of normal human pregnancy. British Journal of Obstetrics and Gynaecology 88: 465–471

Fadel H E, Northop G, Missenheimer R et al 1979 Normal pregnancy: a model of sustained respiratory alkalosis. Journal of Perinatal Medicine 3: 195–201

Hutchon D Jr, Van Zijil J A W M, Campbell-Brown B M, et al 1982 Desmopressin as a test of urinary concentrating ability in pregnancy. Journal of Obstetrics and Gynaecology 2: 206–209

Hytten F E, Cheyne G A 1972 The amino-aciduria of pregnancy. Journal of Obstetrics and Gynaecology of the British Commonwealth 79: 424–432

Hytten F E, Leitch I (eds) 1971 Physiology of human pregnancy, 2nd edn. Blackwell Scientific, Oxford, p 126–128

Lim V S, Katz A I, Lindheimer M D 1976 Acid–base regulation in pregnancy. American Journal of Physiology 231: 1764–1770

Lindheimer N D 1970 Further characterization of the influence of supine posture on renal function. Gynecologic and Obstetric Investigation 1: 69–81

Lindheimer K D, Katz A L 1977 Kidney function and disease in pregnancy. Lea & Febiger, Philadelphia, p 47–76

Lindheimer K D, Katz A L 1985 In: D W Seldin, G Giebisch (eds) The kidney : physiology and pathophysiology. Raven Press, New York, p 2027

Lindheimer M D, Katz A I, Nolten W E et al 1977 Sodium and mineralocorticoid in normal and abnormal pregnancy. Advances in Nephrology 7:33

Lopes-Espinoza I, Dhar H, Humphreys S et al 1986 Urinary albumin excretion in pregnancy. British Journal of Obstetrics and Gynaecology 93:176–181

Nolten W E, Lindheimer M D, Oparil S et al. 1978 Desoxycorticosterone in normal pregnancy. I. Sequential studies of the secretory patterns of desoxycorticosterone, aldosterone and cortisol. American Journal of Obstetrics and Gynecology 132: 414–420

Page E W, Glendening M B, Dignam W et al 1955 The reasons for decreased histidine excretion in preeclampsia. American Journal of Obstetrics and Gynecology 70: 766–773

Pesce A J, First M R 1979 Proteinuria: an integrated review. Marcel Dekker, New York, p 5–31

Pirani B B K, Campbell D A, MacGillvray I 1973 Plasma volume in normal first pregnancy. Journal of Obstetrics and Gynaecology of the British Commonwealth 801: 884–887

Pritchard J A, Barnes A C, Bright R H 1955 The effect of the supine position on renal function in near-term pregnant women. Journal of Clinical Investigation 34: 777–781

Robertson E G 1971 The natural history of oedema during pregnancy. Journal of Obstetrics and Gynaecology of the British Commonwealth 78: 520–529

Robinson M 1958 Salt in pregnancy. Lancet 1: 178–181

Rosenbloom A A, Sach J, Fisher D A 1975 The circulating vasopressinase of pregnancy: species comparison and radioimmunoassay. American Journal of Obstetrics and Gynecology 121: 316–320

Seitchik J, Szutka A, Alper C 1958 Further studies on the metabolism of N^{15}-labeled uric acid in normal and toxaemic pregnant women. American Journal of Obstetrics and Gynecology 76: 1151–1155

Sims E A H, Krantz K E 1958 Serial studies of renal function during pregnancy and the puerperium in normal women. Journal of Clinical Investigation 37: 1764–1774

Thomsen K, Olesen V O 1984 Renal lithium clearance as a measure of the delivery of water and sodium from the proximal tubule in humans. American Journal of the Medical Sciences 288: 158–161

Walters W A W, MacGregor W G, Hills M 1966 Cardiac output at rest during pregnancy and the puerperium. Clinical Science 30: 1–11

Weinberger M H, Kramer N J, Petersen L P et al 1976 Sequential changes in the renin–angiotensin–aldosterone systems and plasma progesterone concentration in normal and abnormal human pregnancy. In: M D Lindheimer, A I Katz, F P Suspan (eds) Hypertension and pregnancy. Wiley, New York, p 263–268

Weir R J, Doig A, Fraser R et al 1976 Studies of the renin–angiotensin–aldosterone system, cortisol DOC, and ADH in normal and hypertensive pregnancy. In: D M Lindheimer, A J Katz, F P Zuspan (eds) Hypertension in pregnancy. Wiley, New York, p 251–260

Welsh G W, Sims E A H. 1960 The mechanisms of renal glucosuria in pregnancy. Diabetes 9: 363–375

4. Pathophysiological mechanisms and pathology in hypertensive disorders of pregnancy

Preeclampsia is the major syndrome among hypertensive disorders of pregnancy in which underlying pathophysiological factors have been intensively studied and debated. There is less interest, indeed less to evoke interest, in the underlying mechanisms when hypertension has been documented before pregnancy in patients with preexisting hypertension or renal disease and where hypertension persists during pregnancy. When superimposed preeclampsia develops in such cases the pathophysiological mechanisms are presumably similar to those operating in preeclampsia.

4.1 GENETIC FACTORS

The familial occurrence of preeclampsia was documented over 100 years ago by Elliot (1873). Elliot reported a fatal case of eclampsia in a family in which a mother and 5 daughters all died of eclampsia.

Chesley et al (1968) carried out an analysis of pregnancies in sisters, daughters, granddaughters and daughters-in-law of patients with eclampsia. They documented a 6% incidence in the daughters-in-law, 37% incidence in sisters and 25% incidence in daughters of patients with preeclampsia, which suggested an autosomal recessive single gene defect in preeclampsia (Chesley 1980). This is further discussed by Chesley & Cooper (1986). Another study demonstrated that preeclampsia was more frequent in mothers but not mothers-in-law of women who had preeclampsia (Sutherland et al 1981). Hypertension in pregnancy has also been reported to be more common in the sisters of women who had hypertensive disorders in their first pregnancy (Adams & Findlayson 1961).

More recently, Arngrimssion et al (1990), in discussing the inheritance of preeclampsia, addressed the possibility of reduced penetrance of a dominant gene.

Redman found an excess of HLA homozygosity in parents of women with preeclampsia and suggested that homozygosity for recessive maternal immune response genes may predispose to severe preeclampsia (Redman et al 1978). Redman seeks to explain the first pregnancy preponderance of preeclampsia by invoking immune mechanisms which induce protection by previous exposure to fetal antigens.

Because of the relation to the HLA system, it has been proposed that the single gene defect in preeclampsia may be located on the short arm of chromosome 6 and much of the current research in this area relates to attempts to clarify this (Anonymous 1988). (References listed at the end of 4.3.)

4.2 BLOOD VOLUME IN HYPERTENSIVE PREGNANCIES

The increased maternal plasma volume seen in normal pregnancy discussed in 3.5.1 is reduced in pregnancies where the baby is small for gestational age (Duffus et al 1971) and in preeclampsia (Cope 1961). In patients with chronic or essential hypertension the plasma volume is also decreased (Gallery et al 1979).

Women with pregnancy associated hypertension retain sodium more avidly than normotensive pregnant women (Chesley et al 1958, Sarles et al 1968) in spite of plasma volume contraction. This sodium retention may be a 'physiological' response to the contracted plasma volume in an attempt to restore it to normal.

Chesley noted the abnormal renal tubular response in hypertensive pregnancies (Chesley et al 1958) and some interest has focused on sodium/potassium ATPase which is the major enzyme involved in active sodium reabsorption by the tubule. This is discussed in 4.3.5.

Increased sensitivity to angiotensin II and increased levels of atrial natriuretic peptide may influence tubular reabsorption of sodium; their interaction is discussed in 4.3.

Despite the marked differences in plasma renin activity, plasma aldosterone concentration, plasma volume and glomerular filtration rate, Brown et al (1988) in a prospective study did not find a difference in sodium excretion between pregnancy and postpartum values. Patients destined to develop preeclampsia had similar sodium excretion to that of normotensive patients in the second trimester. Patients with proteinuric hypertension had the lowest plasma volume, plasma aldosterone concentration and plasma renin activity. These women retained sodium to a similar degree as normotensive women who had been placed on a low sodium diet. Although this study helps to define the relationship between sodium and the renin–aldosterone system, the explanation for the low plasma volume in preeclampsia is not apparent. (References listed at the end of 4.3.)

4.3 VASOACTIVE MECHANISMS AND PREECLAMPSIA

The hypertension of preeclampsia usually develops after 20 weeks' gestation, but there is evidence that in women who do develop preeclampsia the blood pressure is higher in the second trimester than it is in women who do not develop preeclampsia (Fallis & Langford 1963, Page & Christianson 1970, Gallery et al 1977).

Increased or abnormal vascular reactivity was first noted in pregnancy hypertension many years ago. Dieckmann & Michel (1937) reported that the vascular reactivity to vasopressin was increased in preeclampsia compared with normal pregnancy.

There is decreased responsiveness to adrenaline and noradrenaline in normal pregnancy in many species and in pregnant women.

Raab et al (1956) noted that exaggerated pressor responses to adrenaline and noradrenaline may be helpful in predicting preeclampsia, although the test lacked specificity. Mendlowitz noted increased digital reactivity to noradrenaline in midpregnancy in patients destined to develop 'toxaemia' (Mendlowitz 1961). It is generally agreed that the cold pressor test, a simple test of vascular reactivity, has no predictive value for later development of preeclampsia (Chesley & Valenti 1958).

Major interest revolves around the sensitivity to the pressor effects of angiotensin.

Abdul-Karim and Assali (1961) first noted that pregnant women were relatively refractory to the effects of infused angiotensin, and Taledo et al (1968) made the important observation that preeclamptic women were as sensitive to angiotensin as non-pregnant women. Gant et al (1973) described the angiotensin infusion test, which has became the 'gold standard' for predicting which women are destined to develop preeclampsia in later pregnancy on the basis of increased sensitivity to angiotensin (Fig. 4.3.1–1)

Gant subsequently noted that the diastolic blood pressure increased by 20 mmHg or more in women destined to develop preeclampsia when they turned from lateral recumbency to a supine position (Gant et al 1974). The value of this so-called 'roll-over' test in predicting preeclampsia remains controversial (Kassar et al 1980).

In normal pregnancy the circadian rhythm of blood pressure changes is similar to that observed in non-pregnant women showing morning peaks and low pressures at night (Murnaghan et al 1980). In preeclampsia the normal circadian rhythm is reversed, a change which may reflect the influence of hormonal mechanisms controlling the blood pressure.

In addition to catecholamine and angiotensin, many vasoactive substances have been implicated in the pathogenesis of hypertension in pregnancy.

The impact of other pathophysiological mechanisms in preeclampsia is also addressed in later sections.

There has been relatively less interest in some of the hormonal mechanisms which were documented many years ago, namely the increased sensitivity to vasopressin (Dieckman & Michel 1937) and exaggerated pressor responses to adrenaline and noradrenaline (Raab et al 1956).

This chapter will therefore deal mainly with the renin–angiotensin system and its interaction with prostanoids and with some of the newly discovered vasoactive mechanisms involving atrial natriuretic factor, endothelin and endothelium derived relaxing factor now known to be nitric oxide.

4.3.1 The renal angiotensin system and interaction with prostanoids

Since the observation that pregnant women are refractory to angiotensin II infusion (Abdul-Karim & Assali 1961) and the important clinical observation that women destined to develop preeclampsia develop relative increased sensitivity to angiotensin II (Gant et al 1973) (Fig. 4.3.1–1), the renin–angiotensin system has become a major focus of research in this field. More recently, studies have involved the interaction between the renin–angiotensin–aldosterone system and prostaglandins (Fievet et al 1986).

The renin–angiotensin–aldosterone system plays a major role in sodium excretion as well as pro-

ducing vasoconstriction through generation of angiotensin II.

The marked reduction in sensitivity to angiotensin II, which is a characteristic feature of normal pregnancy, is accompanied by an increase in plasma renin activity and plasma renin concentration (Weir et al 1971). By 16 weeks' gestation plasma renin activity and concentration are two to three times that seen in the preovulatory phase (Oats et al 1981) Angiotensin converting enzyme levels increase after 30 weeks' gestation (Oats et al 1981). Plasma aldosterone also shows a marked increase during pregnancy (Chesley 1978, Weir et al 1971).

Plasma angiotensin II levels increase significantly in normal pregnancy, reaching a maximum in the midtrimester; this has been postulated as one mechanism which may be involved in the impaired vascular response to infused angiotensin II. Proponents of this view suggest that the increased sensitivity to angiotensin II which develops in preeclampsia, might result from reduced angiotensin II levels in such patients.

Another hypothesis about the decreased sensitivity to angiotensin II in normal pregnancy is that it may result from increased production of vasodilator prostaglandins. Impaired prostaglandin

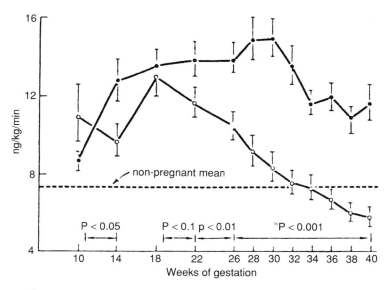

Fig. 4.3.1–1   The amount of angiotensin required to raise the diastolic blood pressure by 20 mmHg in women who subsequently developed preeclampsia (open circles) and in control pregnant women (closed circles). (From Gant et al 1973, with permission.)

production in preeclampsia could then account for the increased sensitivity to angiotensin II in that disorder.

Increased output of endothelium derived relaxing factor has been proposed as another possible factor accounting for decreased angiotensin II sensitivity in normal pregnancy (Nakamato et al 1990).

Reduction in numbers and avidity of vascular angiotensin II receptors are additional features which have been implicated as contributing to the blunted pressor response to angiotensin II in normal pregnancy (Symonds 1988).

More recently, Symonds' group has studied platelet angiotensin II receptors and demonstrated increased angiotensin II binding to platelets in pregnancy induced hypertension (Baker et al 1990a,b). Pawlack & Macdonald (1990) have demonstrated a reduction in platelet angiotensin II receptors in normal pregnancy but not in pregnancy induced hypertension, and believe this may account for the altered angiotensin II responsiveness in preeclampsia.

Of the mechanisms which may be involved in the blunted response to angiotensin II in normal pregnancy there are good data to support the view that prostaglandins participate in this response. Worley et al (1979) studied the dose of angiotensin II (effective pressor dose) required to elevate the diastolic blood pressure by 20 mmHg in pregnant women before and after indomethacin administration. Figure 4.3.1–2 shows that the mean effective pressor dose (EPD A II) required before indomethacin was 20.2 ng/kg/min whereas after indomethacin the sensitivity to angiotensin II was greatly increased and the EPD A II fell to 7.9 ng/kg/min. A similar fall in EPD A II was observed following aspirin administration. It was concluded from this study that, although other mechanisms may be involved, vasodilator prostaglandins (PG) play a pivotal role in the control of vascular tone and angiotensin responsiveness during pregnancy.

Gant's group (Spitz et al 1988) also measured the effect of low dose aspirin on the levels of prostacyclin and thromboxane B_2. Although both decreased, the decrease in thromboxane B_2 was significantly greater than the decrease in the prostacyclin metabolite 6-keto-$PGF_{1\alpha}$ (Spitz et al

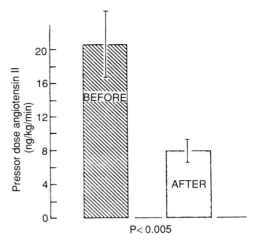

Fig. 4.3.1–2 Dose of angiotensin II required to elevate diastolic blood pressure by 20 mmHg before and after indomethacin administration. (From Worley et al 1979, with permission.)

1988). Effective pressor doses of angiotensin II (EPD A II) are decreased following low dose aspirin in normal pregnant women. In women with preeclampsia and increased sensitivity to angiotensin II, low dose aspirin increased the EPD A II towards that seen in normal pregnant women. Aspirin does not, however, return EPD A II to normal in preeclampsia, and Spitz et al (1988) concluded that the EPD A II reflected only some degree of selective inhibition of thromboxane and not of prostacyclin.

The study by Worley et al (1979), which suggested that vasodilator prostaglandin may be involved in elevation of the blood pressure in pregnancy induced hypertension, was published at a time when several other groups were showing an interest in the involvement of prostacyclin and thromboxane and other prostanoids in preeclampsia. Early studies included those of placental synthesis (Robinson et al 1979) and synthesis in umbilical vessels (Stuart et al 1981, Remuzzi et al 1980) and suggested decreased prostacyclin synthesis and increased thromboxane synthesis in preeclampsia. Subsequent studies of urinary excretion which reflects the 'in vivo' situation in patients with preeclampsia produced some conflicting results. Pedersen et al (1983) reported an increase in PGE_2 excretion in women with preeclampsia, while Fievet et al (1986) found no differences in PGE_2, $PGF_{2\alpha}$ 6-keto-$PGF_{1\alpha}$ or thromboxane levels. The latter authors suggested disarticulation of the renin–prostacyclin loop because of a negative correlation between plasma renin activity and 6-keto-$PGF_{1\alpha}$ in hypertensive pregnant women. Fitzgerald et al (1987) found that prostacyclin metabolite 6-keto-$PGF_{1\alpha}$ excretion was lower in pregnancy hypertension than in normal pregnancies and that this decreased prostacyclin formation could be used to predict later development of hypertension.

More recent studies have supported these findings (Yamaguchi & Mori 1988, Terragno & Terragno 1988) and established that, in addition to a reduction in vasodilator prostaglandin, pregnancy induced hypertension is associated with an increase in thromboxane A_2 synthesis (Fitzgerald et al 1990). This provides a rational basis for the use of aspirin in the prevention and treatment of preeclamspia.

Kallikrein excretion has not been extensively studied. Fievet et al (1986) did not find any differences in kallikrein secretion between normal pregnant women and those with pregnancy induced hypertension. Two other studies have, however, reported lower levels of urinary kallikrein excretion in women with pregnancy induced hypertension (Hiruta et al 1986, Ferrazzani et al 1989).

4.3.2 Endothelin and endothelium derived relaxing factor

It has been suggested that preeclampsia may be an endothelial cell disorder (Roberts et al 1989). There has been considerable interest in the role of endothelin, the newly discovered vasoconstrictor peptide produced by vascular endothelial cells (Yanagiswa et al 1988), in pregnancy induced hypertension.

The powerful vasodilation produced by endothelial cells, through secretion of endothelium derived relaxing factor (EDRF, nitric oxide) has the potential to antagonize the effects of endothelin.

Several recent studies suggest that plasma endothelin-1 levels are increased in preeclampsia (Kamoi et al 1990, Taylor et al 1990, Greer 1991). Branch et al (1991) recently reported that serum from patients with preeclampsia suppresses endothelin production by cultured endothelial cells, but others were unable to confirm this (Brown et al 1991).

Inhibition of EDRF by free haemoglobin has been proposed as one possible mechanism underlying vasoconstriction in preeclampsia (Sarrel et al 1990). Raised free haemoglobin concentrations in preeclampsia, which are related to the intravascular coagulation, correlate with the severity of preeclampsia (Schneider 1951, Pritchard et al 1954), and it has been proposed that this mechanism may play a causal role in vasoconstriction in preeclampsia.

In a study of the in vitro effects of serum from women with preeclampsia, endothelium mediated relaxation was not altered (Tulunko et al 1987). These findings do not support those suggesting that inhibition of EDRF may be involved in the vasoconstriction of preeclampsia.

4.3.3 Atrial natriuretic peptide

Two early studies demonstrated an increase in atrial natriuretic peptide (ANP) secretion in normal pregnancy compared with the non-pregnant state (Thomsen et al 1987, Otsuki et al 1987). In both studies the level of ANP was significantly higher in preeclampsia and pregnancy induced hypertension than in normal pregnancy. Subsequent studies have confirmed these observations (Hirai et al 1988, Bond et al 1989, Fievet et al 1988).

High levels of ANP in pregnancy induced hypertension and preeclampsia correlated with the severity of preeclampsia (Fievet et al 1988, Thomsen et al 1987). ANP levels were not raised in chronic hypertension (Bond et al 1989, Sumioki et al 1989), or in 'toxaemia with oedema only' (Otsuki et al 1987), or in women with proteinuria and oedema without hypertension (Hirai et al 1988). Because of the low plasma volume and low central venous pressure, the high ANP findings in preeclampsia are paradoxical, suggesting that atrial pressure is not a major determinant of ANP levels in preeclampsia.

Plasma ANP levels show a clear-cut circadian rhythm in pregnancy induced hypertension, both mild and severe. This diurnal rhythm is a specific feature of pregnancy induced hypertension (Sumioki et al 1989).

Administration of ANP increases placental blood flow in pregnant rats. In hypertensive rats which had been subjected to 5/6 nephrectomy, ANP doubled the placental blood flow, returning it to normal levels (Chemtob et al 1989).

4.3.4 Serotonin

Serotonin, which is located in platelet dense granules, has been implicated in the hypertension of preeclampsia (Weiner 1987). Serotonin is a powerful vasoconstrictor and is released during platelet aggregation, which is one of the manifestations of intravascular coagulation in preeclampsia (Weiner 1987). Raised serotonin levels reflect platelet aggregation; hence an increase in serum levels could be secondary to platelet aggregation and not imply a primary role in preeclampsia.

4.3.5 Cation transport

The demonstrated abnormalities in vascular reactivity in preeclampsia could be linked to abnormal sodium distribution between intracellular and extracellular compartments. Abnormalities in sodium/potassium ATPase activity were reported in blood from patients with preeclampsia (Kuhnert et al 1977). These were associated with an increased intracellular sodium (Forrester & Alleyne 1980).

Recent studies confirm that the activity of the enzyme sodium/potassium ATPase is significantly reduced in pregnancy induced hypertension and that there is an increase in intracellular sodium (Testa et al 1988, Tranquilla et al 1988).

4.3.6 Calcium

The evidence that there is an inverse relationship between preeclampsia and calcium intake has been reviewed by Belizan et al (1988). It is postulated that a low calcium diet increases parathyroid hormone secretion which leads to increased intracellular calcium and a rise in blood pressure.

A significant rise in platelet calcium levels has been reported in women with preeclampsia (Kilby et al 1990). This was not confirmed in other studies of hypertension in pregnancy (Barr et al 1989); however, the difference could relate to the severity of preeclampsia. Kilby et al (1991) found no increase in platelet calcium levels in non-proteinuric hypertension but found a significant increase in proteinuric preeclampsia.

The potential importance of calcium in preeclampsia has gained considerable impetus from the recent publication of a controlled trial of calcium supplementation in the prevention of preeclampsia. This study by Belizan et al (1991) showed unequivocal benefit from calcium supplementation.

4.3.7 Trace elements

Blood lead (Rabinowitz et al 1987) and zinc (Lazebnik et al 1989) have both been implicated in hypertension during pregnancy.

A high blood lead level correlated with high systolic and diastolic blood pressure levels in pregnancy.

Zinc deficiency has been implicated in hypertension during pregnancy. Both plasma and placental zinc are reported to be lower in women with preeclampsia (Lazebnik et al 1989).

REFERENCES

Abdul-Karim R, Assali N S 1961 Pressor response to angiotensin in pregnant and nonpregnant women. American Journal of Obstetrics and Gynecology 82: 246–251
Adams E M, Finlayson A 1961 Familial aspects of preeclampsia and hypertension in pregnancy. Lancet 2: 1375–1378
Anonymous 1988 Genetics of preeclampsia. Lancet 2: 778
Arngrimsson R, Björnsson S, Geirsson R T et al 1990 Genetic and familial predisposition to eclampsia and preeclampsia in a defined population. British Journal of Obstetrics and Gynaecology 97: 762–769
Baker P N, Pipin F B, Symonds E M 1990a Platelet angiotensin II binding sticks in normotensive and hypertensive pregnancy In: Proceedings VII World Congress of Hypertension in Pregnancy. Perugia, 7–11 October 1990, p 246 (abstract)
Baker P N, Pipkin F B, Symonds E M 1990b Co-linearity between the angiotensin II sensitivity test and platelet AII binding. In: Proceedings VII World Congress of Hypertension in Pregnancy. Perugia, 7–11 October 1990, p 244 (abstract)
Barr S M, Lees K R, Butters L et al 1989 Platelet intracellular free calcium concentration in normotensive and hypertensive pregnancies in the human. Clinical Science 76: 67–71

Belizan J M, Villar J, Repke J 1988 The relationship between calcium intake and pregnancy-induced hypertension: up-to-date evidence. American Journal of Obstetrics and Gynecology 158: 898–902

Belizan J M, Villar J, Gonzalez L et al 1991 Calcium supplementation to prevent hypertensive disorders of pregnancy. New England Journal of Medicine 325: 1399–1405

Bond A L, August P, Druzin M I et al 1989 Atrial natriuretic factor in normal and hypertensive pregnancy. American Journal of Obstetrics and Gynecology 160: 1112–1116

Branch D W, Dudley D J, Mitchell M D 1991 Preliminary evidence for haemostatic mechanism regulating endothelin production in pre-eclampsia. Lancet 337: 843–945

Brown M A, Gallery E D M, Ross M et al 1988 Sodium excretion in normal and hypertensive pregnancy: a prospective study. American Journal of Obstetrics and Gynecology 159: 297–307

Brown M A, Zammit V C, Whitworth J A, et al 1991 Endothelin production in pre-eclampsia. Lancet 338: 261 (letter)

Chemtob S, Potvin W, Varma D R 1989 Selective increase in placental blood flow by atrial natriuretic peptide in hypertensive rats. American Journal of Obstetrics and Gynecology 160: 477–479

Chesley L C, Valenti C, Rein H 1958 Excretion of sodium loads by nonpregnant and pregnant, normal, hypertensive and pre-eclamptic women. Metabolism: Clinical and Experimental 7: 575–588

Chesley L C, Valenti C 1958 The evaluation of tests to differentiate preeclampsia from hypertensive disease. American Journal of Obstetrics and Gynecology 75: 1165–1173

Chesley L C, Annitto J E, Cosgrove R A 1968 The familial factor in toxaemia of pregnancy. Obstetrics and Gynecology 32: 303–311

Chesley L C (ed) 1978 Hypertensive disorders in pregnancy. Appleton-Century-Crofts, New York, p 236

Chesley L C 1980 Hypertension in pregnancy: definitions, familial factor, and remote prognosis. Kidney International 18: 234–240

Chesley L C, Cooper D W 1986 Genetics of hypertension in pregnancy: possible single gene control of preeclampsia and eclampsia in the descendants of eclamptic women. British Journal of Obstetrics and Gynaecology 93: 898–908

Cope I 1961 Plasma and blood volume changes in pregnancies complicated by preeclampsia. Journal of Obstetrics and Gynaecology of the British Commonwealth 68: 413–416

Dieckmann W J, Michel H L 1937 Vascular–renal effects of posterior pituitary extracts in pregnant women. American Journal of Obstetrics and Gynecology 33: 131–137

Duffus G M, MacGillivray I, Dennis K J 1971 The relationship between baby weight and changes in maternal weight, total body water, plasma volume, electrolytes and proteins and urinary oestriol excretion. Journal of Obstetrics and Gynaecology of the British Commonwealth 78: 97–104

Elliot Jr G T 1873 Case 120: puerperal eclampsia in the eighth month: extraordinary family history. Obstetric clinic. Appleton, New York, p 291–293

Fallis N E, Langford H G 1963 Relation of second trimester blood pressure to toxaemia of pregnancy in the primigravid patient. American Journal of Obstetrics and Gynecology 87: 123–125

Ferrazzani S, Leardi P, Magnotti D L et al 1989 Aldosterone, kallikrein, kininase I and II in normal and hypertension complicated pregnancy. Advances in Experimental Medicine and Biology 247B: 455–461

Fievet P, Gregoire I, Brunel P 1986 Renin–angiotensin–aldosterone system, urinary prostaglandin and kallikrein in pregnancy-induced hypertension: evidence for a dysregulation of the renin–angiotensin–prostacyclin loop. Journal of Hypertension 4 (suppl 5): S88–S91

Fievet P, Fournier A, deBold A et al 1988 Atrial natriuretic factor in pregnancy-induced hypertension and preeclampsia: increased plasma concentrations possibly explaining these hypovolaemic states with paradoxical hyporeninism. American Journal of Hypertension 1: 6–21

Fitzgerald D J, Entman S S, Mulloy K 1987 Decreased prostacyclin biosynthesis preceding the clinical manifestation of pregnancy-induced hypertension. Circulation 75: 956–963

Fitzgerald D J, Rocki W, Murray R et al 1990 Thromboxane A_2 synthesis in pregnancy-induced hypertension. Lancet 335: 751–754

Forrester T E, Alleyne G A O 1980 Leucocyte electrolytes and sodium efflux rate constant in the hypertension of preeclampsia. Clinical Science 59: 199–201

Gallery E D M, Ross M, Hunyor S N et al 1977 Predicting the development of pregnancy-associated hypertension. The place of standardized measurement. Lancet 1: 1273–1275

Gallery E D M, Hunyor S N, Gyory A Z 1979 Plasma volume contraction: a significant factor in both pregnancy-associated hypertension (preeclampsia) and chronic hypertension in pregnancy. Quarterly Journal of Medicine 48: 593–602)

Gant N F, Daley G L, Chand S et al 1973 A study of angiotensin II pressor response throughout primigravid pregnancy. Journal of Clinical Investigation 52: 268–269

Gant N F, Chand S, Worley R J et al 1974 A clinical test useful for predicting the development of acute hypertension in pregnancy. American Journal of Obstetrics and Gynecology 120: 1–7

Greer I A, 1991 Endotoxin bound and gagged. Lancet 337: 588–590

Hirai N, Yanaihara Y, Nakayama T et al 1988 Plasma levels of atrial natriuretic peptide during normal pregnancy and in pregnancy complicated by hypertension. American Journal of Obstetrics and Gynecology 159: 27–31

Hiruta M, Furuhashi N, Kono N et al 1986 Urinary kallikrein quantity and activity in patients with pregnancy induced hypertension in third trimester. Clinical and Experimental Hypertension B5(1): 39–50

Kamoi K, Sudo N, Ishibashi M et al 1990 Plasma endothelin-1 levels in patients with pregnancy-induced hypertension. New England Journal of Medicine 323: 1486–1487

Kassar N S, Aldridge J, Quirk B 1980 Roll over test. Obstetrics and Gynecology 55: 411–413

Kilby M D, Pipkin F B, Cockbill S et al 1990 A cross-sectional study of basal platelet intracellular free calcium concentration in normotensive and hypertensive primigravid pregnancies. Clinical Science 78: 75–80

Kilby M D, Pipkin F B, Heptinstall S et al 1991 A comparison of platelet systolic free calcium concentrations in both normotensive and hypertensive primigravidae. In:

Proceedings VII World Congress of Hypertension in Pregnancy. Perugia, 7–11 October; 1990, p 72 (abstract)

Kuhnert B R, Huhnert P M, Murray B A et al 1977 Na/K- and Mg-ATPase activity in the placenta and in maternal and cord erythrocytes of preeclamptic patients. American Journal of Obstetrics and Gynecology 127: 56–60

Lazebnik N, Kuhnert B R, Kuhnert P 1989 Zinc, cadmium, and hypertension in parturient women. American Journal of Obstetrics and Gynecology 16: 437–440

Mendlowitz M, Altchek A, Naftchi N et al 1961 Digital vascular reactivity to L-norepinephrine in the second trimester of pregnancy as a test for latent essential hypertension and toxaemia. American Journal of Obstetrics and Gynecology 81: 643–652

Murnaghan G A, Mitchell R H, Ruff S 1980 Circadian variation of blood pressure in pregnancy. In: Bonnar J, MacGillivray I, Symonds E M (eds) Pregnancy hypertension. MTP Press, Lancaster, p 107–111

Nakamoto D, Hidaka A, Tomoda S et al 1990 Effect of the vascular endothelial cells on refractiveness to angiotensin II of pregnant and non-pregnant rabbits. Significance of EDRF (endothelium -derived relaxing factor) In: Proceedings VII World Congress of Hypertension in Pregnancy. Perugia, 7–11 October 1990 p 163 (abstract)

Oats J N, Pipkin F B, Symonds E M 1981 A prospective study of plasma angiotensin-converting enzyme in normotensive primigravidae and their infants. British Journal of Obstetrics and Gynaecology 88: 1204–1210

Otsuki Y, Okamoto E, Iwata I et al 1987 Changes in concentration of human atrial natriuretic peptide in normal pregnancy and toxaemia. Journal of Endocrinology 114: 325–328

Page E W, Christianson R 1970 The impact of mean arterial pressure in the middle trimester upon the outcome of pregnancy. American Journal of Obstetrics and Gynecology 125: 740–745,

Pawlack M A, MacDonald G J 1990 Possible regulatory disorder of angiotensin II (AII) receptors in pregnancy-induced hypertension (PIH). In: Proceedings VII World Congress of Hypertension in Pregnancy. Perugia, 7–11 October; 1990, p 247 (abstract)

Pedersen E B, Christensen N J, Christensen P et al 1983 Preeclampsia—a state of prostaglandin deficiency? Hypertension 5: 105–111

Pritchard J A, Weisman R, Ratnoff O D et al 1954 Intravascular haemolysis, thrombocytopenia and other haematological abnormalities associated with severe toxaemia of pregnancy. New England Journal of Medicine 250: 89–98

Raab W, Schroeder G, Wagner R et al 1956 Vascular reactivity and electrolytes in normal and toxaemic pregnancy. Journal of Clinical Endocrinology and Metabolism 16: 1196–1216

Rabinowitz M, Bellinger D, Leviton A et al 1987 Pregnancy hypertension, blood pressure during labor, and blood lead levels. Hypertension 10: 447–451

Redman C W G, Bodner J G, Godner W F et al 1978 Preeclampsia/antigens in severe preeclampsia. Lancet 2: 397–399

Remuzzi G, Marchesi D, Zoja C et al 1980 Reduced umbilical and placental vascular prostacyclin in severe preeclampsia. Prostaglandins 20: 105–110

Roberts J M, Taylor R N, Musci T J et al 1989 Preeclampsia: an endothelial cell disorder. American Journal of Obstetrics and Gynecology 161: 1200–1204

Robinson J S, Redman C W G, Clover L et al 1979 The concentrations of the prostaglandins E and F, 13, 14-dihydro-15 oxoprostaglandin F and thromboxane B1 in tissues obtained from women with and without pre-eclampsia. Prostaglandins and Medicine 3: 223–234

Sarles H E, Hill S S, LeBlanc A L et al 1968 Sodium excretion patterns during and following intravenous sodium chloride loads in normal and hypertensive pregnancies. American Journal of Obstetrics and Gynecology 102: 1–7

Sarrel P M, Lindsay D C, Poole-Wilson P A et al 1990 Hypothesis: inhibition of endothelium-derived relaxing factor by haemoglobin in the pathogenesis of pre-eclampsia. Lancet 2: 1030–1032

Schneider C L 1951 Fibrin embolism (disseminated intravascular coagulation) and the aetiology of eclampsia. Journal of Obstetrics and Gynaecology of the British Empire 58: 538–554

Spitz B, Magness R R, Cox S M et al 1988 Effect on angiotensin II pressor responses and blood prostaglandin concentrations in pregnant women sensitive to angiotensin II. American Journal of Obstetrics and Gynecology 159: 1035–1043

Stuart M J, Sunderji S G, Yambo T et al 1981 Decreased prostacyclin production: a characteristic of chronic placental insufficiency syndromes. Lancet 1: 1126–1128

Sumioki H, Shimokawa H, Miyamoto S et al 1989 Circadian variations of plasma atrial natriuretic peptide in four types of hypertensive disorder during pregnancy. British Journal of Obstetrics and Gynaecology 96: 922–927

Sutherland A, Cooper D W, Howie P W et al 1981 The incidence of severe preeclampsia amongst mothers and mothers-in-law of preeclamptics and controls. British Journal of Obstetrics and Gynaecology 88: 785–791

Symonds E M 1988 Renin and reproduction. American Journal of Obstetrics and Gynecology 158: 754–761

Taledo O E, Chesley L C, Zuspan F P 1968 Renin–angiotensin system in normal and toxaemic pregnancies. III. Differential sensitivity to angiotensin II and norepinephrine in toxaemia of pregnancy. American Journal of Obstetrics and Gynecology 100: 218–221

Taylor R N, Varma M, Teng N N H et al 1990 Women with preeclampsia have higher plasma endothelin levels than women with normal pregnancies. Journal of Clinical Endocrinology and Metabolism 71: 1675–1677

Terragno N A, Terragno A 1988 Mechanisms of hypertension in pregnancy. Seminars in Nephrology 8: 138–146

Testa I, Rabini R A, Danieli G et al 1988 Abnormal membrane cation transport in pregnancy-induced hypertension. Scandinavian Journal of Clinical and Laboratory Investigation 48: 7–13

Thomsen J K, Storm T L, Thamsborg G et al 1987 Atrial natriuretic peptide concentrations in preeclampsia. British Medical Journal 294: 1508–1510

Tranquilla A L, Mazzanti L, Bertoli E et al 1988 Sodium/potassium -adenosine triphosphatase on erythrocyte ghosts from pregnant women and its relationship to pregnancy-induced hypertension. Obstetrics and Gynecology 71: 627–630

Tulunko T, Schneider J, Floro C et al 1987 The in vitro effect on arterial wall function of serum from patients with pregnancy-induced hypertension. American Journal of Obstetrics and Gynecology 56: 817–823

Weiner C P 1987 The role of serotonin in the genesis of

hypertension in preeclampsia. American Journal of Obstetrics and Gynecology 156:885-888

Weir R J, Paintin D B, Brown J J et al 1971 A serial study in pregnancy of the plasma concentrations of renin, corticosteroid, electrolytes and proteins: and of haematocrit and plasma volume. Journal of Obstetrics and Gynaecology of the British Commonwealth 78: 590-602

Worley R J, Gant N F, Everett R B et al 1979 Vascular responsiveness to pressor agents during human pregnancy. Journal of Reproductive Medicine 23: 115-128

Yamaguchi M, Mori N 1988 Urinary excretion of 6-ketoprostaglandin $F_{1\alpha}$ in preeclampsia. Archives of Gynecology and Obstetrics 244: 7-13

Yanagiswa M, Kurihara H, Kimura S et al 1988 A novel potent vasoconstrictor peptide produced by vascular endothelial cells. Nature 332: 411-415

4.4 COAGULATION ABNORMALITIES IN PREGNANCY INDUCED HYPERTENSION AND PREECLAMPSIA

Normal pregnancy is associated with increased blood levels of coagulation factors (Stirling et al 1984) and suppression of fibrinolysis (Wiman et al 1984). The increased risk of thromboembolism in pregnancy has been attributed to these changes (De Boer et al 1989).

In 1890 Pilliet described ectatic dilatation of capillaries in the liver filled with spherical thrombi in eclampsia, and shortly afterwards Schmorl (1893) described hyaline and fibrin thrombi in glomerular capillaries in this condition.

This evidence of intravascular coagulation in preeclampsia and eclampsia described 100 years ago has been confirmed in many subsequent studies. Intravascular coagulation is thought to account for many, perhaps all, of the generalized manifestations of eclampsia and preeclampsia. Thus the proteinuria is associated with fibrin deposits in the kidneys while microthrombi in the brain and liver may well be major factors in the cerebral manifestations of eclampsia and the liver disturbances in this condition.

The so-called HELLP syndrome, in which there is haemolytic anaemia, liver enzyme abnormalities and thrombocytopenia, is one of the more serious clinical syndromes associated with preeclampsia and is essentially due to disseminated intravascular coagulation.

The defibrination syndrome seen in association with abruptio placentae (Schneider 1951) is one end of the spectrum of coagulation–fibrinolysis abnormalities seen in pregnancy.

At the other end of the spectrum in early preeclampsia, the only abnormalities in coagulation noted may be a decreased platelet count and raised levels of fibrin degradation products in the serum (Jespersen 1980).

The fact that aspirin may correct both the platelet count and high levels of fibrin degradation products (Jespersen 1980) as well as improving the clinical manifestations of preeclampsia (Crandon & Sherwood 1979) suggests that coagulation abnormalities may play a primary role in the causation of eclampsia and preeclampsia.

Page (1948) and Schneider (1951) introduced the concept of intravascular coagulation as one of the pathogenetic mechanisms in preeclampsia. Morris et al (1964) identified fibrin in glomeruli using antifibrinogen antiserum and were among the first to investigate the coagulation and fibrinolytic systems in preeclampsia. McKay et al (1953) described the features of disseminated intravascular coagulation at autopsy. Pritchard et al (1954) documented intravascular haemolysis, thrombocytopenia and other coagulation abnormalities in patients with severe toxaemia. Brakman & Astrup (1963) in an early study reported significant inhibition of fibrinolysis in late normal pregnancy, and much of the more recent interest in coagulation disorders in preeclampsia relates to an increase in plasminogen activator inhibitor levels in preeclampsia (De Boer et al 1988, Estelles et al 1989).

Coagulation abnormalities demonstrated in preeclampsia include thrombocytopenia (Howie et al 1976, Boneu et al 1980, Gibson et al 1982), increased factor XII and decreased factor X and factor XI (Lox et al 1983, Conde 1976), and increased fibrinogen (Chatergee et al 1978, McKilop et al 1976). These abnormalities reflect a consumptive coagulopathy or disseminated intravascular coagulation and support a primary role for the coagulation mechanism in preeclampsia (Sher et al 1975, Roberts & May 1976, Bonner et al 1976, Imrie & Raper 1977, Conde 1976). Activation of the intrinsic coagulation pathway has been proposed as the mechanism underlying some of these abnormalities (Redman 1979, Vaziri et al 1986).

A recent detailed study of the haemostatic system in preeclampsia (Saleh et al 1987) demonstrated high fibronectin levels, low antithrombin III levels and low α2-antiplasmin, suggesting a combination of endothelial injury and fibrinolysis. Saleh (1987) proposed the model illustrated in Figure 4.4–1 to explain the abnormalities seen in preeclampsia. Ballegeer (1989) also stressed the value of fibronectin levels in predicting gestational hypertension.

Saleh et al (1987) also reported an increase in platelet volume — a change confirmed by others (Rosevear & Liggins 1986, Walker et al 1989) and one which probably reflects increased platelet turnover as young platelets are large. They did not find evidence of thrombocytopenia, which has been documented in several previous studies (Burrows 1990, Romero et al 1989), perhaps

because they studied patients just before and after delivery when levels return towards normal. Burrows (1990) found the overall risk of thrombocytopenia in hypertensive patients to be 13%, but found that this was greatly influenced by the stage of gestation and no greater than the thrombocytopenia found in a control population beyond 37 weeks of gestation.

There are many studies documenting low antithrombin III levels in preeclampsia (Kiobayashi & Terao 1987, Gilabert et al 1988, Friedman et al 1986, Hayakawa & Maki 1988, Lieberman et al 1988, Weenink et al 1984, De Boer et al 1989). Several authors have also reported increased fibrin degradation products (Trofatter et al 1989, Beller et al 1979, Kiobayashi & Terao 1987) and attributed these to a chronic state of disseminated intravascular coagulation.

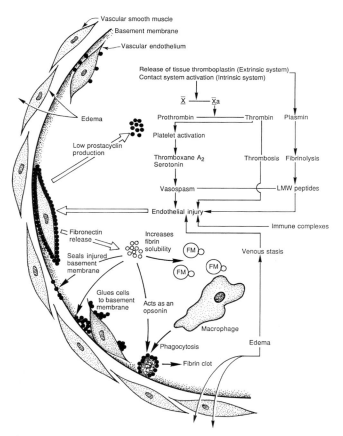

Fig.4.4–1 A model for the effects of pregnancy induced hypertension (preeclampsia) on the haemostatic system. Note the central role of endothelial injury. LMW peptides refers to low molecular weight fibrinolytic peptides. FM, fibrin monomer. (From Saleh et al 1987, with permission.)

Recent studies have focused on defects in the fibrinolytic system which may account for fibrin deposition in preeclampsia. Tissue plasminogen activator, which converts plasminogen to plasmin, is a key fibrinolytic enzyme. The activity of tissue plasminogen activator is regulated by plasminogen activator inhibitor (PAI). The levels of PAI increase progressively in normal pregnancy and a further increase in PAI activity has been noted in preeclampsia (Aznar et al 1986, Estelles et al 1987, De Boer et al 1988). More recent studies suggest that type 1 plasminogen activator inhibitor (PAI-1) accounts for the high plasma PAI activity in severe preeclampsia and that PAI-1 levels correlate with the severity of placental damage (Estelles et al 1989). These authors suggested that the abnormal placenta may be the source of the increased PAI-1 but that part of the increased PAI-1 may originate from platelets which are activated in preeclampsia. The prominence of fibrin deposition in the pathological lesions of preeclampsia has led to the use of heparin (Bonnar et al 1976, Whitworth & Fairley 1973), antithrombin III concentrate (Teroa 1989) and aspirin and thromboxane synthetase inhibitors (Beaufils et al 1985) in the treatment or prevention of preeclampsia.

Much of the recent interest in the antithrombotic agents dipyridamole and aspirin (Beaufils et al 1985, 1986) in the prevention and treatment of preeclampsia stems from the observation of thrombotic lesions and intravascular coagulation in preeclampsia.

The abnormalities in coagulation in preeclampsia cannot be divorced from the abnormalities in vasoactive mechanisms discussed in 4.3. Prostanoids, in addition to being powerful vasoconstrictors and vasodilators, play an important role in coagulation mechanisms.

Correlations between the kallikrein–renin system and coagulation abnormalities have been noted (Hayakawa & Maki 1988), and other vasoactive substances such as angiotensin, endothelin and EDRF all interact with the coagulation system at the endothelial level.

Although antiendothelial antibodies have been demonstrated in preeclampsia (Raidt 1985) there has been surprisingly little interest in this area.

Other factors which may contribute to intra-vascular coagulation, such as increased blood viscosity (Zondervan et al 1988) and reduced erythrocyte filterability (Rodgers et al 1988), have not been extensively studied. The latter abnormality may be more important in pregnancies in diabetic women.

Platelet membrane fluidity is said to be reduced in pregnancy induced hypertension (Gleeson et al 1990) and this could be an additional factor which predisposes to platelet aggregation.

REFERENCES

Aznar J, Gilabert J, Estelles A et al 1986 Fibrinolytic activity and protein C in preeclampsia. Thrombosis and Haemostasis 55: 314–317

Ballegeer V, Spitz B, Kieckens L et al 1989 Predictive value of increased plasma levels of fibronectin in gestational hypertension. American Journal of Obstetrics and Gynecology 165: 432–436

Beaufils M, Uzan S, Donsimoni R et al 1985 Prevention of preeclampsia by early anti-platelet therapy. Lancet 1: 1–3

Beaufils M, Uzan S, Donsimoni R et al 1986 Prospective controlled study of early antiplatelet therapy in prevention of preeclampsia. Advances in Nephrology 15: 87–94

Beller F K, Ebert C H, Dame W R 1979 High molecular fibrin derivatives in pre-eclamptic and eclamptic patients. European Journal of Obstetrics, and Gynecology, and Reproductive Biology 105–110

Boneu B, Fournie A, Sie P et al 1980 Platelet production time, uremic, and some haemostasis tests in preeclampsia. European Journal of Obstetrics, Gynecology, and Reproductive Biology 11: 85–94

Bonnar J, Redman C W G, Denson K W 1976 The role of coagulation and fibrinolysis in preeclampsia. In: M D Lindheimer, A I Katz , F P Zuspan (eds) Hypertension in pregnancy. Wiley, New York, p 85–93

Brakman P, Astrup T 1963 Selective inhibition in human pregnancy blood of urokinase induced fibrinolysis. Scandinavian Journal of Clinical and Laboratory Investigation 15: 603–609

Burrows R F 1990 Thrombocytopenia in the hypertensive disorders of pregnancy. Clinical and Experimental Hypertension Part B Hypertension in Pregnancy B9: 199–209

Chatergee T, Maitra D, Chakravfty T et al 1978 Studies on plasma fibrinogen level in preeclampsia and eclampsia. Experientia 34: 562–563

Conde R G 1976 A serial study of coagulation factors XII, XI, and X in plasma in normal pregnancy and in pregnancy complicated by preeclampsia. British Journal of Obstetrics and Gynaecology 83: 636–639

Coopland A T 1969 Blood clotting abnormalities in relation to pre-eclampsia: a review. Canadian Medical Association Journal 100: 121–124

Crandon A J, Isherwood D M 1979 Effect of aspirin on incidence of preeclampsia. Lancet 1: 1356

De Boer K, Lecander I, ten Cate J W et al 1988 Placental-type plasminogen activator inhibitor in preeclampsia. American Journal of Obstetrics and Gynecology 158: 518–522

De Boer K, ten Cate J W, Sturk A et al 1989 Enhanced thrombin generation in normal and hypertensive pregnancy. American Journal of Obstetrics and Gynecology 160: 95–100

Estelles A, Gilabert J, Espana F et al 1987 Fibrinolysis in preeclampsia. Fibrinolysis 1: 209

Estelles A, Gilabert J, Asner J et al 1989 Changes in the plasma levels of Type 1 and Type 2 plasminogen activator inhibitors in normal pregnancy and in patients with severe preeclampsia. Blood 74: 1332–1338

Friedman K D, Borok Z, Owen J 1986 Heparin co-factor activity and antithrombin III antigen levels in preeclampsia. Thrombosis Research 43: 409–416

Gibson B, Hunder D, Neame P B et al 1982 Thrombocytopenia in preeclampsia and eclampsia. Seminars in Thrombosis and Hemostasis 8: 234–237

Gilabert J, Fernandes J A, Espana F et al 1988 Physiological coagulation inhibitors (Protein S, Protein S, Protein C and Antithrombin III) in severe preeclamptic states and in users of oral contraceptives. Thrombosis Research 49: 319–329

Gleeson R, Ahmen Y, Rice-Evans C et al 1990 Platelet membrane fluidity in pregnancy hypertension. Lancet 335: 225–226

Hayakawa M, Maki M 1988 Coagulation–fibrinolytic and kinin-forming systems in toxaemia of pregnancy. Gynecologic and Obstetric Investigation 26: 181–190

Howie P W, Purdie D W, Begg C B et al 1976 Use of coagulation tests to predict the clinical progress of preeclampsia. Lancet 2: 323–325

Imrie A H, Raper C G 1977 Severe intravascular coagulation preceding severe preeclampsia. British Journal of Obstetrics and Gynaecology 84: 71–72

Jespersen J 1980 Disseminated intravascular coagulation in toxaemia of pregnancy. Correction of the decreased platelet counts and raised levels of serum uric acid and fibrin(ogen) degradation products by aspirin. Thrombosis Research 17: 743–746

Kiobayashi T, Terao T 1987 Preeclamspia as chronic disseminated intravascular coagulation. Gynecologic and Obstetric Investigation 24: 170–178

Lieberman J R, Hagay Z J, Mozoi M et al 1988 Plasma antithrombin III levels in preeclampsia and chronic hypertension. International Journal of Gynaecology and Obstetrics 27: 21–24

Lox C D, Dorsett M M, Hampton R M 1983 Observations on clotting activity during preeclampsia. Clinical and Experimental Hypertension 2: 179–190

McKay D G, Merrill S J, Weiner A E et al 1953 The pathological anatomy of eclampsia, bilateral renal cortical necrosis, pituitary necrosis and other acute fatal outcomes of pregnancy and its possible relationship to the generalized Schwartzmann reaction. American Journal of Obstetrics and Gynecology 66: 507–539

McKilop C, Forbes C D, Howie P W et al 1976 Soluble fibrinogen/fibrin complexes in preeclampsia. Lancet 2: 56–58

Morris R H, Vassali P, Beller F K et al 1964 Immunofluorescent studies of renal biopsies in diagnosis of toxaemia of pregnancy. Obstetrics and Gynecology 24: 32

Page E W 1948 Heparin and toxaemia of pregnancy. Obstetrical and Gynecological Survey 3: 615

Pilliet A 1890 Nouvelles recherches sur le foi des eclamptiques. Nouvelles Archives d'Obstetriques 5: 600–607

Pritchard J A, Weisman R, Ratnoff O D et al 1954 Intravascular haemolysis, thrombocytopenia and other haematolytic abnormalities associated with severe toxaemia of pregnancy. New England Journal of Medicine 250: 89–98

Raidt 1985 In: C. Goecke (ed) Actual standing in EPH-gestosis. Elsevier, Amsterdam, p 313–317

Redman C W 1979 Coagulation problems in human pregnancy. Postgraduate Medical Journal 55: 367–371

Roberts J M, May W J 1976 Consumptive coagulopathy in severe preeclampsia. Obstetrics and Gynecology 48: 163–166

Rodgers B D, Hreshchyshyn M M, Lee R V et al 1988 Erythrocyte filterability in normal and high-risk pregnancy. Obstetrics and Gynecology 71: 192–197

Romero R, Mazor M, Lockwood C J et al 1989 Clinical significance, prevalence, and natural history of thrombocytopenia in pregnancy-induced hypertension. American Journal of Perinatology 6: 32–38

Rosevear S K, Liggins G C 1986 Platelet dimensions in pregnancy-induced hypertension. New Zealand Medical Journal 26: 356–357

Saleh A A, Bottoms S F, Welch R A et al 1987 Preeclampsia, delivery and the haemostatic system. American Journal of Obstetrics and Gynecology 157: 331–336

Schmorl G 1893 Pathologisch-anatomische Untersuchungen uber puerperal Eklampsie. Leipzig

Schneider C L 1951 'Fibrin embolism' (disseminated intravascular coagulation) with defibrination as one of the end results during placenta abruptio. Surgery, Gynecology and Obstetrics 92: 27–34

Sher G, Davey D A, Ogilvie M et al 1975 Pregnancy, Pre-eclampsia and disseminated intravascular coagulation. South African Medical Journal 49: 1197–1200

Stirling Y, Woolf L, North W R et al 1984 Haemostasis in normal pregnancy. Thrombosis and Haemostasis 52: 176–182

Teroa T, Kobayashi T, Imai N et al 1989 Pathological state of the coagulatory and fibrinolytic system in preeclampsia and the possibility of its treatment with AT III concentrate. Asia–Oceania Journal of Obstetrics and Gynaecology 15: 25–32

Trofatter K F, Howell M L, Greenberg C S, et al 1989 Use of the fibrin D-dimer in screening for coagulation abnormalities in preeclampsia. Obstetrics and Gynecology 73: 435–439

Vaziri N D, Toohey J, Powers D et al 1986 Activation of intrinsic coagulation pathway in preeclampsia. American Journal of Medicine 80: 103–107

Walker J J, Cameron A D, Bjornsson S et al 1989 Can platelet volume predict progressive hypertensive disease in pregnancy? American Journal of Obstetrics and Gynecology 161: 676–679

Weenink G H, Treffers P E, Vijn P et al 1984 Antithrombin II levels in preeclampsia correlate with maternal and fetal morbidity. American Journal of Obstetrics and Gynecology 148: 1092

Whitworth J A, Fairley K F 1973 Heparin in the treatment of preeclamptic toxaemia. In: P Kincaid-Smith, T H Mathew, E Becker (eds) Glomerulonephritis. Wiley, New York, p 1027

Wiman B, Csemiczky G, Marsk L et al 984 The fast-acting inhibitor of tissue plasminogen activator in plasma during pregnancy. Thrombosis and Haemostasis 52: 124–126

Zondervan H A, Oosting J, Smorenberg-Schoorl M E, et al 1988 Maternal whole blood viscosity in pregnancy hypertension. Gynecologic and Obstetric Investigation 25: 83–88

4.5 MORPHOLOGICAL CHANGES IN PREECLAMPSIA

4.5.1 Morphological changes in placental vessels in pregnancy hypertension

The morphological changes in placental vessels assume particular significance because the vascular abnormalities characteristic of preeclampsia develop at a very early stage in pregnancy. The waves of trophoblast invasion of uterine vessels which are abnormal in preeclampsia are complete by 16 weeks of gestation; hence the scene is set as early as 16 weeks for the development of the typical vascular lesions in the placenta in preeclampsia and for the later clinical manifestations of this syndrome.

The critical observations of the morphological changes in uteroplacental vessels which constitute the physiological response to pregnancy reported by Brosens et al (1967) and their detailed analysis in relation to the abnormalities characteristic of preeclampsia (Robertson et al 1967, 1975, 1976) are consistent with the functional data of Gant et al (1973) that the abnormal vascular reactivity characteristic of preeclampsia develops at a very early stage of gestation long before clinical manifestations appear.

This very early development of both the abnormal vascular reactivity and the abnormal morphological lesions has very important implications for the prevention of preeclampsia, indicating that treatment needs to start very early if it is to prevent the disease process of preeclampsia. It may be possible to reverse the functional changes at a later stage but the morphological changes in the uteroplacental vessels are clearly irreversible from very early in pregnancy, although they may undergo some subsequent modification.

The importance of placental ischaemia as an underlying mechanism in preeclampsia and the observation of placental infarcts associated with preeclampsia (Bartholomew & Kracke 1932) led to detailed studies of placental vessels. These revealed so called acute atherosis of decidual vessels in preeclampsia (Bartholemew & Kracke 1936). Many subsequent studies have confirmed these changes (Hertig 1945).

Distinctive changes, labelled as acute atherosis by Zeek & Assali (1950), are characteristic of the vascular damage in the placental bed in preeclampsia.

Perhaps the most distinctive feature of the lesions of acute atherosis is the presence of numerous large mononuclear foam cells. Although this is a feature of experimental atheroma (Leary 1941), it is also a lesion seen in other conditions where acute thrombosis occurs in blood vessels — for example, in acute allograft rejection (Kincaid-Smith 1975a). The foam cells are characteristically seen during 'organization' of intravascular thrombus and fibrin.

Since the recognition of placental vascular abnormalities 50 years ago, there has been confusion between the physiological lesions which occur in the uteroplacental blood supply and the superimposed pathological lesions of preeclampsia. This confusion was clarified by the major contribution of Robertson et al (1967, 1975, 1976) which clearly distinguished the different morphological components in preeclampsia and hypertension from the striking physiological changes which occur in placental vessels. In normal pregnancy trophoblast invades the decidual portion of the spiral arteries at an early stage. At 12–16 weeks this trophoblast 'invasion' extends into the myometrial segments of the spiral arteries (Fig. 4.5.1–1). As part of these changes, much of the vessel wall is replaced by fibrinoid material and vessels undergo progressive enlargement due to distension of their walls. In the fully developed stage of physiological change, the media has been replaced by 'fibrinoid' material and inflammatory cells and giant cells surround the vessel wall. The radial and arcuate arteries are not affected by these changes nor are the basal arteries which remain normal.

In preeclampsia the essential difference from the normal physiological change is the failure of trophoblast invasion into the myometrial segment of the spiral artery. This results in a narrow segment of the spiral artery as well as relative narrowing of the decidual portion of the spiral artery (Fig. 4.5.1–2).

Acute atherosis, a lesion in which the media of the vessel is replaced by fibrinoid necrosis and the intima is lined by fibrin and lipid laden macrophages or smooth muscle cells, is a pathognomonic change in preeclampsia. It affects myo-

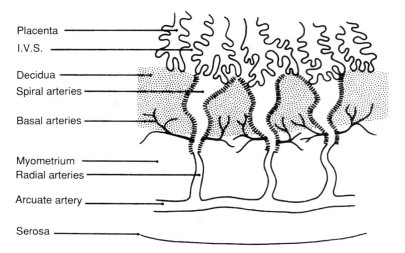

Fig. 4.5.1–1   Diagrammatic representation of the fully developed physiological changes in the uteroplacental arteries in normal pregnancy. The hatched portions of the walls of these vessels indicate the extent of the physiological changes. Note that the basal arteries represented by solid black outlines are unaffected by these changes. (From Robertson et al 1976, with permission.)

metrial segments of spiral arteries that have not undergone so-called 'physiological' changes — the termination of spiral arteries in the decidua and in the basal arteries. The decidual segments of uteroplacental arteries which have already undergone physiological changes associated with invasion by trophoblast and distension of the vessel wall appear to be immune from the effects of so-called acute atherosis in patients with preeclampsia (Fig. 4.5.1–3).

There can be no doubt that the acute arterial lesions of preeclampsia account for the increased thrombosis and placental infarction seen in preeclampsia. These vascular lesions are also the morphological counterpart of the markedly re-duced uteroplacental blood flow in preeclampsia (Lunell et al 1982).

While acute atherosis is the most characteristic lesion of preeclampsia, some degree of hypertensive arteriosclerosis of myometrical segments of the spiral artery is also seen, particularly in women who have preexisting hypertension — either essential hypertension or hypertension associated with renal disease. In the fully developed form of this hypertensive arteriosclerosis, the arterial wall undergoes fibrinoid necrosis (Robertson et al 1975).

A further point of significance in our understanding of preeclampsia is that a similar inadequate maternal vascular response to placen-

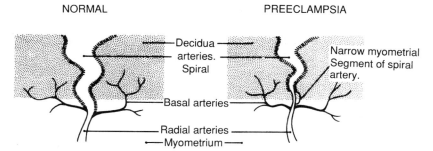

Fig. 4.5.1–2   Diagram showing the difference between normal and preeclamptic pregnancies in the extent of physiological changes in the uteroplacental arteries. Note that in preeclampsia these changes do not extend beyond the deciduomyometrial junction leaving a constricting segment of the placental bed spiral arteries between the parent radial arteries and the decidual portions of the uteroplacental arteries. (From Robertson et al 1976, with permission.)

Preeclampsia: atherosis (O)

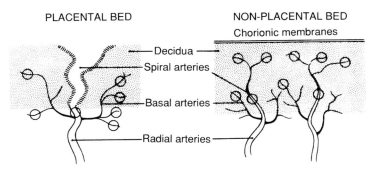

Fig. 4.5.1–3   Tomography of acute atherosis in preeclampsia. Note that the lesions occur in segments of vessels unaffected by physiological changes in the placental bed (left) and in the decidua vera (right). (From Robertson et al 1976, with permission.)

tation with failure of trophoblast to invade many placental bed arteries occurs in pregnancies which result in infants that are small for gestational age (Khong et al 1986).

4.5.2   Renal pathology in preeclampsia

The kidney is so obviously involved in the major clinical manifestations of preeclampsia that older pathologists registered some surprise at the relative absence of renal lesions in fatal cases of eclampsia.

Schmorl (1901) first described fibrin and hyaline thrombi in glomeruli in three cases of fatal eclampsia. Thrombi had previously been described in liver vessels when Pillet (1880) described 'une grappe de raisin' — spherical thrombi in ectatic blood vessels in the liver in preeclampsia.

In the kidney, the presence of preexisting vascular lesions and glomerular disease may complicate the pathological lesions which occur in preeclampsia. Zimmerman & Peters (1937) were probably the first to point to the frequency of underlying renal disease in patients with so-called pregnancy toxaemia. They noted vascular lesions of malignant nephrosclerosis as a frequent finding in this series and pointed to the discrepancy between the 'benign' clinical features of hypertension during pregnancy in some of the patients who showed malignant nephrosclerosis at autopsy. These might have been cases of thrombotic microangiopathy developing during pregnancy (further discussed in 6.3.3 and 7.2).

Hey Groves (1902) may have been referring to glomerular lesions of thrombotic microangiopathy in his reference to the hyaline thrombi which occur in eclampsia in association with anaemia. He compared the lesions with glomerular thrombi seen in swine cholera, which is a form of thrombotic microangiopathy. He also noted positive staining with Weigert's fibrin dye, a good method of identifying fibrin (Kincaid-Smith et al 1958).

Glomerular lesions of eclampsia/preeclampsia

Although it is agreed by all that the glomerular capillary lumen is reduced and glomeruli are bloodless, there are different views about the nature of the lesions causing narrowing of glomerular capillaries. Early workers (Lohlein 1918, Fahr 1928, Bell 1932, Baird & Dunn 1933) all noted thickening of the glomerular capillary wall as the major abnormality. Bell used azocarmine stains to distinguish between the basement membrane and endothelial and epithelial cells and concluded that, 'When the azocarmine stain is applied to the glomerulus in eclampsia, it is easily seen that the thickening of the capillary wall is due, almost entirely, to a massive thickening of the basement membrane'. Lohlein (1918) and Bell (1932) described swelling of glomerular epithelial cells, and Bell's description of hyaline droplets in these cells was probably the first description of this characteristic lesion (Hill et al 1988). Lohlein (1918), Fahr (1928), Bell (1932), Baird & Dunn (1933) all described an increase in number and swelling of endothelial (or intracapillary) cells. Fahr attributed this to an infectious process. A strong message comes through from these pathologists, each of whom was an acknowledged expert in his field, that there was an unequivocal increase in thickness of the capillary wall; they placed rather less emphasis on the contribution of swelling of the endothelial cell to this process. Endotheliosis, which is often regarded as the pathognomonic feature of preeclampsia (Spargo et al 1959), attracted less attention from earlier pathologists, perhaps because Spargo's was an ultrastructural study and the endothelial cell is both better defined and more prominent on electron microscopy than on light microscopy. While it is well accepted that so-called endotheliosis is part of the glomerular picture of preeclampsia, it is not an isolated lesion but occurs in conjunction with many other lesions including subendothelial deposits, basement membrane changes and epithelial cell changes.

There are undoubtedly some cases of preeclampsia in which the major abnormality appears to be a thickening of the glomerular capillary wall itself. One such case is illustrated in Figure 4.5.2–1 and resolution of the changes 2 months later in Figure 4.5.2–2. In this case the thickening of the glomerular capillary wall is clearly due to subendothelial deposits of fibrin or fibrinoid material which have disappeared in the biopsy done 2 months later and can therefore be attributed to the preeclampsia. These are presumably the capillary wall changes described by Lölein (1918) and Fahr (1928), and demonstrated particularly by Bell (1932) with azocarmine stain. They correspond to subendothelial deposits which are often prominent on electron micrographs (Fig. 4.5.2–3).

It is noteworthy that the capillary wall changes illustrated in Figure 4.5.2–1 and Figure 4.5.2–3 which consist of subendothelial fibrin deposits hardly merit a mention in Spargo's 1959 description of endotheliosis, or in a much more recent description of glomerular lesions of preeclampsia (Spargo et al 1976). In this paper subendothelial deposits were not mentioned on light microscopy and in only 7 of 30 specimens were small deposits observed on electron microscopy.

Hopper et al (1961) on the other hand, described subendothelial deposits in all 3 cases of preeclampsia/eclampsia and these were seen in all glomeruli and in 1 case in every capillary. Thomson et al (1972) in a study of 33 women with preeclampsia found subendothelial deposits similar to those illustrated in Figure 4.5.2–3 'as equally

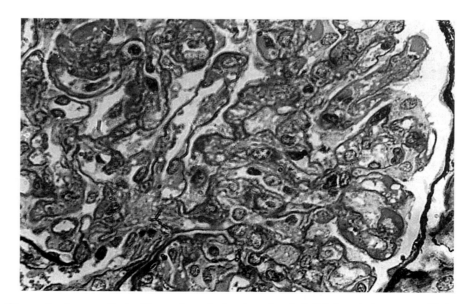

Fig. 4.5.2–1   Glomerulus from a patient with preeclampsia showing subendothelial deposits in many capillaries.

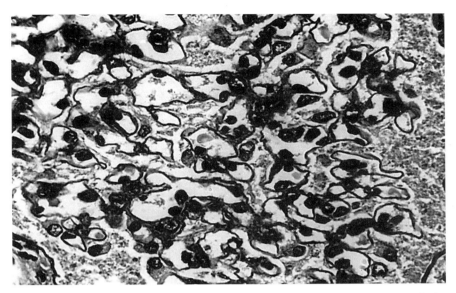

Fig. 4.5.2–2   Glomerulus from a biopsy in the same patient as illustrated in Figure 4.5.2–1 taken 2 months later and showing disappearance of the subendothelial deposits.

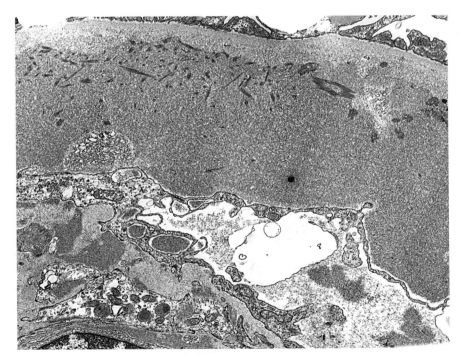

Fig. 4.5.2–3   Electron micrograph from a patient with severe preeclampsia showing a large subendothelial deposit containing fibrillar fibrin.

consistent' to those of endothelial cell swelling and we would concur with that view. Pirani et al (1963), on the other hand, found fibrinoid sub-

endothelial deposits in only 2 of 8 patients with preeclampsia. Endothelial swelling has been noted in all descriptions of the changes of preeclampsia

(Hopper et al 1961, Pirani et al 1963, Fisher et al 1969).

Because the timing of the renal biopsy differs in different studies we explored this as one of the possible explanations for prominence of subendothelial deposits in some studies and the fact that they are hardly mentioned in others. We suspected from our own observations in serial biopsies that subendothelial deposits are rapidly reabsorbed in the early postpartum period. Where subendothelial deposits were consistently noted, as in the study by Thomson et al (1972), the biopsies were done in the first few postpartum days.

On the basis of a blind morphometric analysis, we found that a significant reduction in subendothelial deposits occurs in the early postpartum period (Figures 4.5.2–4 and 4.5.2–5) (Packham et al 1988, Kincaid-Smith 1991). As the subendothelial deposits disappear, the percentage of the glomerular capillary occupied endothelial cells increases and endothelial changes become more prominent (Packham et al 1988).

The rapid alteration in the lesion seen in the glomerular capillary in the first few postpartum days may well explain the differences in observations of different pathologists quoted above. A study based on biopsies carried out 8–10 days after delivery would rarely show subendothelial deposits but would show large prominent endothelial cells.

A further change in endothelial cells related to and perhaps best regarded as a part of so-called 'endotheliosis' is the presence of foam cells in glomeruli. Spargo et al (1976) found foam cells in almost all cases of preeclampsia and described the lesion as part of endotheliosis. Seymour et al (1976) also frequently found foam cells (35% of cases). Seymour's biopsies were carried out up to 12 days postpartum while the timing of Spargo is not stated. We rarely see foam cells in biopsies performed during pregnancy or in the immediate postpartum period. This is in accord with Sheehan's experience in which he documented foam cells in only 4% of autopsies in women who died during pregnancy but in 18% of those who died after delivery. We believe that foam cells are phagocytic macrophages similar to those seen in the placenta in acute atherosis. They are seen in

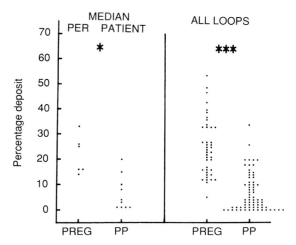

Fig. 4.5.2–4 Morphometric analysis of subendothelial deposits in glomerular capillaries in biopsies taken during pregnancy and in the postpartum period (PP). Both the median measurement of the percentage of the glomerular capillary occupied by deposit (*P<0.05) and the percentage of capillary occupied by deposits in all capillary loops (***P<0.001) are significantly reduced in the postpartum period.

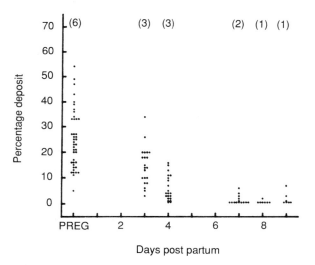

Fig.4.5.2–5 Percentage of capillary six occupied by subendothelial deposit in six biopsies taken during pregnancy from patients with preeclampsia compared with the percentage of the capillary occupied by deposit in the postpartum period (PP). By 6 days postpartum subendothelial deposits have disappeared.

glomeruli in many conditions associated with resolution of thrombotic and fibrinoid lesions. Similar cells are seen in biopsies in malignant hypertension scleroderma and in graft rejection, particularly while fibrin is resolving during treatment (Kincaid-Smith 1975a).

Another component of the capillary wall, namely the basement membrane, also undergoes striking changes in preeclampsia, some of which persist for months after pregnancy. Although considerable remodelling of the basement membrane occurs (Sheehan 1950) perhaps the most obvious and significant change is a reduplication of basement membrane (Fig. 4.5.2–6). Double contours enclose subendothelial deposits and mesangial cell interposition is seen within these deposits (Kincaid-Smith 1973a, 1975b) (Fig. 4.5.2–7). The changes may very closely mimic those seen in mesangio-capillary glomerulonephritis with subendothelial deposits. Deposits disappear within days of delivery, basement membrane changes and reduplication may resolve rapidly after pregnancy, but in individual cases may persist for months (Fig. 4.5.2–6) (Kincaid-Smith 1975b). Typical chain-like lesions of the basement membrane are seen in some cases (Fig. 4.5.2–8) (Kincaid-Smith 1975a). Accompanying this remodelling of the basement membrane of the glomerular capillary wall, there is an increase in laminin, type IV collagen, fibronectin and basement membrane proteoglycan (Foidart et al 1983).

The epithelial cell also participates in the changes which occur in the glomerular tuft in preeclampsia. Epithelial cells are large and characteristically contain prominent hyaline droplets (Fig. 4.5.2–9). These were previously noted by Bell (1932) and by Sheehan (1980).

The percentage of glomeruli in which epithelial cell droplets are seen correlates with the grade of preeclampsia (Kincaid-Smith et al 1985). The composition of the droplets as defined by immunoelectron microscopy is shown in Table 4.5.2–1. Within individual droplets, an outer less dense area, as well as an inner dense core, can be defined on electron microscopy. Fibrinogen staining is usually confined to the inner dense core, whereas immunoglobulins, particularly IgM, are often confined to the outer less dense zone (Fig. 4.5.2–10) (Kincaid-Smith 1991).

Vassalli et al (1963), in describing several biopsies from women with preeclampsia, made a strong case for a pathogenetic role for fibrin in the glomerular lesion of preeclampsia. Strong positive staining with antifibrinogen serum was present in all 11 biopsies, whereas none was found

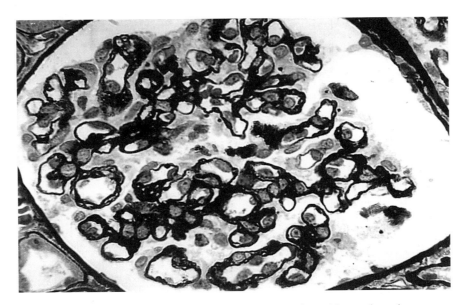

Fig. 4.5.2–6   Double contours in glomerular capillaries in a biopsy from a patient with preeclampsia.

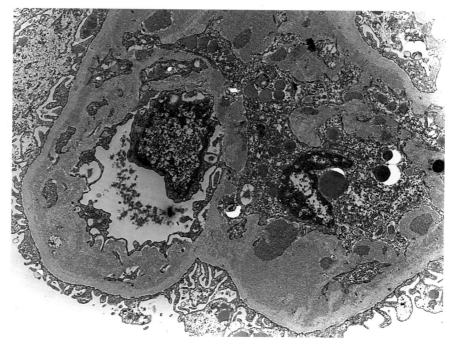

Fig. 4.5.2–7   Electron micrograph showing mesangial cell interposition in subendothelial deposits in preeclampsia.

in a series of control biopsies, and subsequent studies have confirmed that fibrinogen staining is usually present in preeclampsia (Seymour et al 1976). On electron microscopy prominent fibrillar fibrin can be identified within dense subendothelial deposits (Fig. 4.5.2–3).

The glomerular lesions of preeclampsia resemble the lesions of intravascular coagulation.

One confusing aspect of the glomerular lesions of preeclampsia is their relation to the lesion of focal and segmental hyalinosis.

The lesions of preeclampsia may be almost identical to those first described by Habib in the childhood nephrotic syndrome as 'hyalinosis focal et segmentaire'. (Habib et al 1961, Habib 1970). Figure 4.5.2–11 shows a glomerular lesion from a

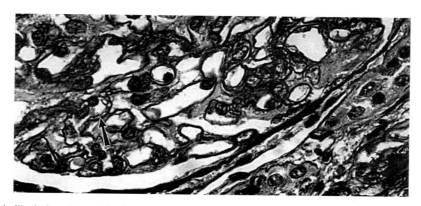

Fig. 4.5.2–8   Chain like lesions (arrow) in glomerular capillaries in a biopsy from a woman with preeclampsia.

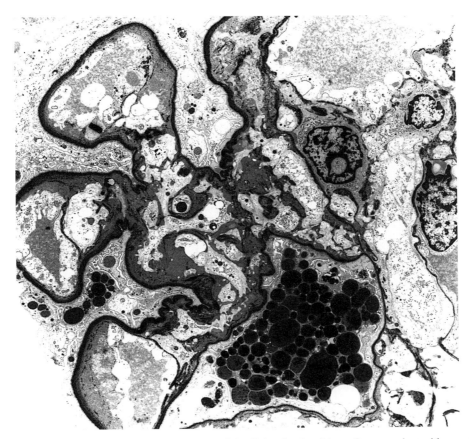

Fig.4.5.2–9   Electron micrograph showing prominent epithelial cell droplets in a biopsy from a patient with preeclampsia.

patient with preeclampsia which is virtually indistinguishable from the lesion of focal and segmental hyalinosis seen in the nephrotic syndrome. Inability to distinguish between these lesions and the lesion of preeclampsia first became apparent to us in 1962, when lesions similar to those illustrated in Figure 4.5.2–11 were noted in pregnancy, and attributed to preeclampsia in a patient who,

after the pregnancy, developed rapidly progressive focal and segmental hyalinosis leading to renal failure (Kincaid-Smith et al 1967, Kincaid-Smith & Fairley 1987).

Recently three other groups have made reference to lesions of focal and segmental hyalinosis and sclerosis developing during preeclampsia (Kida et al 1985, Nochy et al 1986, Gaber & Spargo 1987).

Table 4.5.2–1 Relationship between immunolabelling pattern of glomerular droplets in visceral epithelial cells and mesangial cells (from Kincaid-Smith 1991, with permission)

Case examined	Area examined	IgA	IgG	IgM	C_3c	Fib	Alb
_Preeclamptic toxaemia	Visceral C(P)	+(+)	+(+)	+(+)	+(+)	++(−)	+++(+++)
	Deposit	+	+	+++	+	+++	+
Preeclamptic toxaemia	Mesangial C(P)	−(+++)	−(+++)	−(+++)	+(+)	+++(−)	++(+++)
	Deposit	+	+	+++	+	+++	+

C(P), glomerular cell droplet, core area (peripheral zone); Deposit, adjacent intraglomerular deposit; Fib, fibrinogen; Alb, albumin.

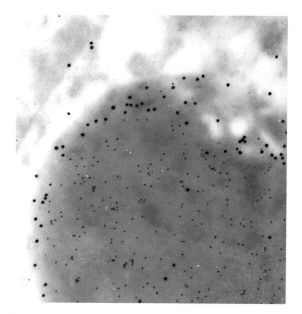

Fig. 4.5.2–10   Hyaline droplet in epithelial cell using double labelling with immunogold particles showing smaller particles, labelling fibrin in the centre of the particles, labelling IgM in the peripheral zone of the droplet. (From Kincaid-Smith 1991, with permission.)

Gaber & Spargo (1987) suggest that the focal sclerosis, as they call it, is of an ischaemic nature and is part of the hypertensive process. They found vascular lesions in 5 of 7 cases and regarded the focal segmental glomerulosclerosis as an indicator of underlying nephrosclerosis and not as part of preeclampsia.

We would favour the view that lesions of focal and segmental hyalinosis and sclerosis, because they may be indistinguishable from lesions of pure preeclampsia, represent one of the variations in the lesions which can be regarded as a manifestation of preeclampsia. They must be distinguished from the lesions of underlying primary or secondary focal and segmental hyalinosis where this is possible.

Arterial and arteriolar lesions in the kidney in preeclampsia

McKelvey & MacMahon (1935) drew attention to vascular lesions in the kidney in patients with pregnancy toxaemias. They described lesions of malignant nephrosclerosis in a group of women

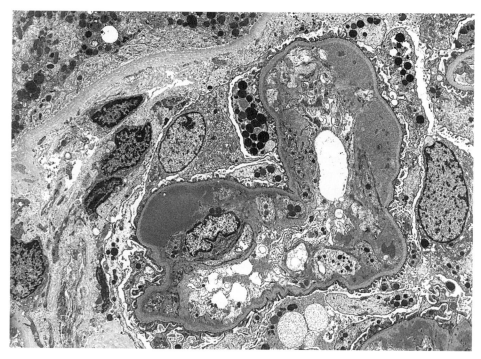

Fig. 4.5.2–11   Ultrastructure of a glomerular capillary in a patient with preeclampsia. The lesions consist of a large vacuolated subendothelial 'fibrinoid' deposit; it is indistinguishable from the lesion of segmental hyalinosis, the key lesion in focal sclerosis of glomerulonephritis.

in whom it appeared that toxaemia of pregnancy produced permanent vascular damage and caused death in a short period of time. All the patients described by McKelvey & MacMahon had pre-existing hypertension.

Zimmerman & Peters (1937) also described vascular lesions of malignant hypertension in women who died of eclampsia/preeclampsia and pointed to the disparity between benign hypertension clinically with malignant vascular lesions at autopsy.

We described fulminating malignant hypertension and anuria in 3 young women who had not had hypertension prior to pregnancy (Kincaid-Smith et al 1958). The vascular lesions in these young women seemed inappropriate in relation to the blood pressure levels and in retrospect they were almost certainly cases of thrombotic micro-angiopathy with renal failure (discussed in 6.3).

Since renal biopsies have become available, prominent and often inappropriate vascular lesions have been noted in women presenting with pre-eclampsia; 14 of 66 biopsies from multiparas with no anaemia showed 'findings characteristic of nephrosclerosis' on renal biopsy (Dieckmann et al 1958). In another early study, 10 of 59 young primiparous women who presented with toxaemia of pregnancy showed renal arteriolar disease (Smythe et al 1964).

We have documented the development of vascular lesions during pregnancies associated with preeclampsia in women with and without underlying renal disease (Kincaid-Smith 1973). Such vascular lesions may appear during pregnancy in patients who do not become hypertensive (Kincaid-Smith & Fairley 1976). Fisher et al (1981) documented nephrosclerosis in 50% of multigravid women in a biopsy study of women with pre-eclampsia. The mean age of these women was 22.5 years and these lesions therefore clearly cannot be attributed to essential hypertension which is very rare at that age.

Vascular lesions, commonly inappropriate in relation to the age of the patients and the level of blood pressure, are a prominent feature in biopsies from women who have had hypertension during pregnancy. Although milder in degree, they have been likened to the thrombotic microangiopathy associated with postpartum renal failure (Kincaid-

Smith 1973b). In women with a circulating lupus anticoagulant, striking vascular lesions may develop during pregnancy, particularly in pregnancies prolonged beyond 16–20 weeks (Kincaid-Smith et al 1988).

REFERENCES

Baird D, Dunn J S 1933 Renal lesions in eclampsia and nephritis of pregnancy. Journal of Pathology and Bacteriology 37: 291–307

Bartholomew R A, Kracke R R 1932 The relation of placental infarcts to eclamptic toxaemia. American Journal of Obstetrics and Gynecology 24: 797–819

Bartholomew R A, Kracke R R 1936 The probable role of the hypercholesteraemia of pregnancy in producing vascular changes in the placenta, predisposing to placental infarction and eclampsia. American Journal of Obstetrics and Gynecology 31: 549–562

Bell E T 1932 Renal lesions in the toxaemias of pregnancy. American Journal of Pathology 8: 1–41

Brosens I, Robertson W B, Dixon H G 1967 The physiological response of the vessels of the placental bed to normal pregnancy. Journal of Pathology and Bacteriology 93:569

Dieckmann W J, McCartney C P, Harrod J P 1958 Kidney biopsies in multiparous patients with vascular renal disease in pregnancy. American Journal of Obstetrics and Gynecology 75: 634–655

Fisher E R, Pardo V, Paul R et al 1969 Ultrastructural studies in hypertension. American Journal of Pathology 55: 109–131

Fisher K A, Luger A, Spargo B H et al 1981 Hypertension in pregnancy: clinical-pathological correlations and remote prognosis. Medicine 60: 267–276

Foidart J M, Nochy B, Nusgens J B et al 1983 Accumulation of several basement membrane proteins in glomeruli of patients with preeclampsia and other hypertensive syndromes of pregnancy. Laboratory Investigation 49: 250–259

Fahr Th 1928 Uber die Nierenveranderungen bei der Eklampsie und ihre Abgrenzung gegen andere Formen des Morbus Brightii. Zentralblatt fur Gynakologie 52: 474–480

Gaber L W, Spargo B H 1987 Pregnancy-induced nephropathy: the significance of focal segmental glomerulosclerosis. American Journal of Kidney Diseases 9: 317–323

Gant N F, Daley G L, Chand S et al 1973 A study of angiotensin II pressor response throughout primigravid pregnancy. Journal of Clinical Investigation 52: 268–289

Habib R 1970 Classification anatomique des nephropathies glomerulaires. Paediatrische Fortbildungskurse fuer die Praxis 28: 3–47

Habib R, Michielsen P, De Montera H et al 1961 Clinical microscopic and electron microscopic data in the nephrotic syndrome of unknown origin. In: Wolstenholme G E W, Cameron M P (eds) Renal biopsy. Ciba Foundation Symposium, J. & A. Churchill, London, p 70–92

Hertig A T 1945 Vascular pathology in hypertensive albuminuric toxaemias of pregnancy. Clinics 4: 602–614

Hey Groves E W 1902 The pathology and treatment of puerperal eclampsia, with special reference to the use of saline transfusion (with notes of two cases). Transactions of the Obstetric Society of London 43: 118–142

Hill P A, Fairley K F, Kincaid-Smith P et al 1988 Morphologic changes in the renal glomerulus and the juxtaglomerular apparatus in human preeclampsia. Journal of Pathology 156: 291–303

Hopper J, Farquhar M G, Yamauchi H et al 1961 Renal lesions in pregnancy. Obstetrics and Gynecology 17: 271–293

Khong T Y, De Wolf F, Robertson W B et al 1986 Inadequate maternal vascular response to placentation in pregnancies complicated by pre-eclampsia and by small-for-gestational age infants. British Journal of Obstetrics and Gynaecology 93: 1049–1059

Kida H, Takeda S, Yokoyama H et al 1985 Focal glomerular sclerosis in preeclampsia. Clinical Nephrology 24: 221–227

Kincaid-Smith P 1973a The role of coagulation in the obliteration of glomerular capillaries. In: P Kincaid-Smith, T H Mathew, E L Becker (eds) Glomerulonephritis. Wiley, New York, p 871–890

Kincaid-Smith P 1973b The similarity of lesions and underlying mechanism in preeclamptic toxaemia and post-partum renal failure. Studies in the acute stage and during follow-up. In: P Kincaid-Smith, T H Mathew, E L Becker (eds) Glomerulonephritis. Wiley, New York, p 1013–1025

Kincaid-Smith P (ed) 1975a The kidney — a clinicopathological study. Blackwell Scientific, Oxford, p 42, 305

Kincaid-Smith P 1975b Participation of intravascular coagulation in the pathogenesis of glomerular and vascular lesions. Kidney International 7: 242–253

Kincaid-Smith P 1991 Renal lesion of preeclampsia revisited. American Journal of Kidney Diseases 17: 144–148

Kincaid-Smith P, Fairley K F 1976 In: M D Lindheimer, A I Katz, F P Zuspan (eds) Hypertension in pregnancy. Wiley, New York, p 157–167

Kincaid-Smith P, Fairley K F 1987 Renal disease in pregnancy. Three controversial areas: mesangial IgA nephropathy, focal glomerular sclerosis (focal and segmental hyalinosis and sclerosis), and reflux nephropathy. American Journal of Kidney Diseases 9: 328–333

Kincaid-Smith P, McMicheal J, Murphy E A 1958 The clinical course and pathology of hypertension with papilloedema (malignant hypertension). Lancet 1: 508–509

Kincaid-Smith P, Fairley K F, Bullen M 1967 Kidney disease and pregnancy. Medical Journal of Australia 2: 1155–1159

Kincaid-Smith P, North R A, Becker G J et al 1985 Proteinuria during pregnancy. In: V E Andreucci (ed) The kidney in pregnancy. Martinus Nijhoff, Boston, p 133–164

Kincaid-Smith P, Fairley K F, Kloss M 1988 Lupus anticoagulant associated with renal thrombotic microangiopathy and pregnancy related renal failure. Quarterly Journal of Medicine 69: 795–815

Leary T 1941 Genesis of atherosclerosis. Archives of Pathology 32: 507–555

Lohlein M 1918 Zur Pathogenese der Nierenkrankheiten. Deutsche Medizinische Wochenschrift 44: 1187

Lunell N O, Nylund L E, Lewander R et al 1982 Uteroplacental blood flow in preeclampsia measurements with indium–113m and a computer-linked gamma camera. Clinical and Experimental Hypertension 1: 105–117

McKelvey J L, MacMahon H E 1935 A study of the lesions in the vascular system in fatal cases of chronic nephritic toxaemia of pregnancy. Surgery, Gynecology and Obstetrics 60: 1–18

Mautner W, Churg J, Grishman E et al 1962 Preeclamptic nephropathy. Laboratory Investigation 11: 518–530

Nochy D, Nihglais N, Jacquot C et al 1986 De novo focal glomerulosclerosis in preeclampsia. Clinical Nephrology 25: 1–85

Packham D K, Mathews D S, Fairley K F et al 1988 Morphometric analysis of preeclampsia in women biopsied in pregnancy and post partum. Kidney International 34: 704–711

Pillet 1880 Gazette Hebdomadaire de Médecine et de Chirugie P 349

Pirani C L, Pollak W E, Lannigan R et al 1963 The renal glomerular lesions of preeclampsia: Electron microscopic studies. American Journal of Obstetrics and Gynecology 87: 1047–1070

Robertson W B, Brosens I, Dixon G 1967 The pathological response of the vessels of the placental bed to hypertensive pregnancy. Journal of Pathology and Bacteriology 93: 581–592

Robertson W B, Brosens I, Dixon G 1975 Uteroplacental vascular pathology. European Journal of Obstetrics, Gynecologys and Reproductive Biology 5: 47–65

Robertson W B, Brosens I, Dixon G 1976 Maternal uterine vascular lesions in the hypertensive complications of pregnancy. In: M D Lindheimer, A Katz, F P Zuspan (eds) Hypertension in pregnancy. Wiley, New York, p 115–127

Schmorl G 1901 Zur Lehre von der Eklampsie. Archiv fur Gynakologie p 504–529

Seymour A E, Petrucco O M, Clarkson A R et al (eds) 1976 In: Hypertension in pregnancy. Wiley, New York, p 139–154

Sheehan H L 1980 Renal morphology in preeclampsia. Kidney International 18: 241–252

Smythe C M, Bradham W S, Dennis E J et al 1964 Renal arteriolar disease in young primiparas. Journal of Laboratory and Clinical Medicine 63: 562–573

Spargo B, McCartney C P, Winemiller R 1959 Glomerular capillary endotheliosis in toxaemia of pregnancy. Archives of Pathology 68: 593–599

Spargo B H, Lichtig C, Luger A M et al 1976 In: Lindheimer M D, Katz A, Zuspan F P (eds) Hypertension in pregnancy. Wiley, New York, p 129–197

Thomson D, Paterson W G, Smart G E et al 1972 The renal lesions of toxaemia and abruptio placentae studied by light and electron microscopy. The Journal of Obstetrics and Gynaecology of the British Commonwealth 79: 311–320

Vassalli P, Morris R H, McCluskey RT 1963 The pathogenic role of fibrin deposition in the glomerular lesions of toxaemia of pregnancy. Journal of Experimental Medicine 118: 467–478

Zeek P M, Assali N S 1950 Vascular changes in the decidua associated with eclamptogenic toxaemia of pregnancy. American Journal of Clinical Pathology 20: 1099–1109

Zimmerman H M, Peters J P 1937 Pathology of pregnancy toxaemias. Journal of Clinical Investigation 16: 397–420

5. Hypertensive disorders of pregnancy

Hypertension develops in some 10% of all pregnancies and is more common in first pregnancies and multiple pregnancies.

5.1 CLASSIFICATION OF HYPERTENSIVE DISORDERS OF PREGNANCY

The three most widely used classifications of hypertensive disorders of pregnancy are the WHO classification (WHO Study Group 1987), the classification proposed by the American College of Obstetrics and Gynecology (ACOG) in 1972, which was recently adopted by the NIH Working Group Report on High Blood Pressure in Pregnancy (1990), and the more detailed classification of Davey & MacGillivray (1988) which was based on their earlier publication (Davey & MacGillivray 1986) adopted by the International Society for the Study of Hypertension in Pregnancy.

The WHO classification (Table 5.1–1) and the classification proposed by Davey & MacGillivray (Table 5.1–2) are both far more detailed and comprehensive than the ACOG classification and allow any patient presenting during pregnancy to be included under one or other specific category.

The NIH working group on high blood pressure in pregnancy argued in favour of the practical and concise nature of the ACOG classification which has only four categories:

1. Chronic hypertension
2. Preeclampsia
3. Preeclampsia superimposed on chronic hypertension and
4. Transient hypertension

A major defect in the ACOG classification is the fact that it excludes a relatively large group of patients who have underlying chronic renal disease rather than underlying chronic hypertension and who develop superimposed preeclampsia. In a renal biopsy study 22% of a consecutive series of women presenting with hypertension in pregnancy had underlying renal disease (Fisher et al 1981). It should also be recognized that many women with underlying renal disease do not develop hypertension during pregnancy.

Although the number of categories in the three classifications are very different, the definitions are essentially similar. A diastolic blood pressure of 90 mmHg or above is the diagnostic criterion of gestational hypertension used by the WHO study group, and a blood pressure of 140/90 is the level used by ACOG. It is worth noting that Browne (Browne & Dodds 1942) suggested that a blood pressure over 130/70 before 20 weeks gestation should be regarded as 'hypertension'.

An increase in blood pressure levels is an important criterion in the diagnosis of preeclampsia particularly because of the fall in blood pressure which occurs in early pregnancy. Unless one takes note of an increase in blood pressure a definition based on 140/90 will certainly exclude some cases of preeclampsia. The ACOG classification notes the importance of an increase in blood pressure levels in its definition of preeclampsia (systolic blood pressure increase of 30 mmHg or diastolic blood pressure increase of 15 mmHg).

There has been a recent proposal for an important change in the definition of preeclampsia in relation to the rise observed in diastolic blood pressure (Redman & Jefferies 1988). On the basis of an analysis of 16 211 singleton pregnancies, Redman & Jefferies proposed that the definition of preeclampsia should include a first diastolic

Table 5.1–1   WHO Classification (from 'The hypertensive disorders of pregnancy' WHO 1987)

1. Gestational hypertension — hypertension without the development of significant proteinuria (<0.3 g/ℓ):
   a. After 20 weeks of gestation;
   b. During labour and/or within 48 h of delivery.
2. Unclassified hypertension in pregnancy — hypertension found when blood pressure is recorded for the first time:
   a. After 20 weeks of gestation;
   b. During labour and/or within 48 h of delivery.
   This type of hypertension should be reclassified as gestational postnatal period, although some of these patients may have underlying hypertension caused by renal disease.
3. Gestational proteinuria — development of significant proteinuria (≥0.3 g/ℓ):
   a. After 20 weeks of gestation;
   b. During labour and/or within 48 h of delivery.
4. Preeclampsia — development of gestational hypertension and significant proteinuria:
   a. After 20 weeks of gestation;
   b. During labour and/or within 48 h of delivery.
5. Eclampsia:
   a. Antepartum;
   b. Intrapartum;
   c. Postpartum.
6. Underlying hypertension or renal disease (for example, in women who initially have hypertension only during pregnancies, being normotensive between pregnancies, but develop sustained hypertension later in life):
   a. Underlying hypertension;
   b. Underlying renal disease;
   c. Other known causes of hypertension (such as phaeochromocytoma).
7. Preexisting hypertension or renal hypertension and/or proteinuria in pregnancy (for example, in women known to have disease prior to pregnancy):
   a. Preexisting hypertension;
   b. Preexisting renal disease;
   c. Preexisting other known causes of hypertension.
8. Superimposed preeclampsia/eclampsia:
   a. Preexisting hypertension with superimposed preeclampsia or eclampsia (a worsening of hypertension, with an increase in diastolic blood pressure to at least 15 mmHg (2.0 kPa) above non-pregnancy values, accompanied by the development or worsening of proteinuria);
   b. Preexisting renal disease with superimposed preeclampsia or eclampsia.
   The terms superimposed preeclampsia and eclampsia should be used only when hypertension was known to be present prior to pregnancy, or when hypertension is discovered early in pregnancy and proteinuria develops in late pregnancy.

blood pressure below 90 mmHg, a subsequent increase of at least 25 mmHg and a maximum reading of at least 90 mmHg. These criteria were applied to a second set of 15 624 pregnancies and successfully identified those with preeclampsia. These new criteria excluded women with mild 'chronic' hypertension.

In defining superimposed preeclampsia the WHO classification accepts an increase of diastolic blood pressure of 15 mmHg above prepregnancy values. In practice an increase of 15 mmHg above levels in the first 20 weeks is almost certainly a more sensitive method of detecting preeclampsia and many cases could be excluded if the increase were related to prepregnancy blood pressure levels which are usually higher than those in the first trimester. Women who are hypertensive before pregnancy have an even greater decrease in blood pressure in pregnancy than do normotensive women

(Chesley & Annitto 1947) and thus the comparison with prepregnancy blood pressures seems inappropriate.

Clearly all these classifications have some merit and some disadvantages both in categories of gestational hypertension and in their definition.

One of the most contentious issues is the recent recommendation from the NIH working group that the Korotkoff V not Korotkoff IV should be used (NIH 1990) in measuring diastolic blood pressure. It has been traditional to use Korotkoff phase IV and this was recommended by the WHO study group because in some 15% of women Korotkoff V or disappearance of the sound is found at 0 mmHg (WHO Study Group 1987). Davey & MacGillivray (1988) also favoured the conventional view that Korotkoff phase IV or muffling of the sound should be taken as the measurement of the diastolic blood pressure measurement. A working

Table 5.1–2   Clinical classification of hypertensive disorders of pregnancy (from Davey & MacGillivray 1988 with permission)

A. Gestational hypertension and/or proteinuria
Hypertension and/or proteinuria developing during pregnancy, labour, or the puerperium in a previously normotensive non-proteinuric woman subdivided into
  1. Gestational hypertension (without proteinuria)
    a. Developing antenatally
    b. Developing for the first time in labour
    c. Developing for the first time in the puerperium
  2. Gestational proteinuria (without hypertension)
    a. Developing antenatally
    b. Developing for the first time in labour
    c. Developing for the first time in the puerperium
  3. Gestational proteinuria hypertension (preeclampsia)
    a. Developing antenatally
    b. Developing for the first time in labour
    c. Developing for the first time in the puerperium
B. Chronic hypertension and chronic renal disease
Hypertension and/or proteinuria in pregnancy in a woman with chronic hypertension or chronic renal disease diagnosed before, during, or after pregnancy subdivided into
  1. Chronic hypertension (without proteinuria)
  2. Chronic renal disease (proteinuria with or without hypertension)
  3. Chronic hypertension with superimposed preeclampsia
    Proteinuria developing for first time during pregnancy in a woman with known chronic hypertension
C. Unclassified hypertension and/or proteinuria
Hypertension and/or proteinuria found either
  1. At first examination after twentieth week of pregnancy (140 days) in a woman without known chronic hypertension or chronic renal disease
or

  2. During pregnancy, labour, or the puerperium where information is insufficient to permit classification is regarded as unclassified during pregnancy and is subdivided into
    1. Unclassified hypertension (without proteinuria)
    2. Unclassified proteinuria (without hypertension)
    3. Unclassified proteinuric hypertension
D. Eclampsia
The occurrence of generalized convulsions during pregnancy, during labour, or within 7 days of delivery and not caused by epilepsy or other convulsive disorders

Notes on classification:
A. Hypertension and/or proteinuria at the first visit before the twentieth week of pregnancy (in the absence of trophoblastic disease) is presumed to be caused by either
  1. Chronic hypertension (hypertension only)
or

  2. Chronic renal disease (proteinuria with or without hypertension)
B. Unclassified hypertension and/or proteinuria may be reclassified after delivery
  1. If the hypertension and/or proteinuria disappears into
    a. Gestational hypertension (without proteinuria)
or

    b. Gestational proteinuria (without hypertension)
or

    c. Gestational proteinuric hypertension (preeclampsia)
  2. If the hypertension and/or proteinuria persists after delivery or other tests confirm the diagnosis into
    a. Chronic hypertension (without proteinuria)
or

    b. Chronic renal disease (proteinuria with or without hypertension)
or

  3. Chronic hypertension with superimposed preeclampsia
C. Gestational proteinuric hypertension may be regarded as synonymous with 'preeclampsia'. 'Gestational hypertension' is often regarded as synonymous with 'pregnancy-induced hypertension', but the term 'pregnancy-induced hypertension' is reserved in this classification for that form of hypertension that commonly but not exclusively occurs in primigravid women and is primarily caused by an abnormality of pregnancy, which if it is severe or progresses is associated with the development of proteinuria and other features of 'preeclampsia.'

party in Australia currently preparing a consensus statement on hypertension in pregnancy also favours the use of Korotkoff phase IV.

Disappearance of a sound is easier to detect than muffling of a sound, and there may be some virtue in recording both the muffling and the disappearance of the sound, but most groups clearly favour the use of Korotkoff IV for use in defining hypertension in pregnancy.

Other factors which need to be considered are the posture of the patient and the cuff size.

Blood pressures taken in the sitting position are generally used and differ little from those taken in a lateral recumbent position provided that the arm is at the level of the heart.

The most frequent error in choosing a cuff is that a standard cuff is used when the arm diameter is too large. If the arm diameter is more then 33 cm a large cuff (15 cm x 33 cm) should be used.

REFERENCES

American College of Obstetrics and Gynecology 1986 Management of preeclampsia. ACOG Technical Bulletin No. 91

Browne F J, Dodds G H 1942 Pregnancy in the patient with chronic hypertension. Journal of Obstetrics and Gynaecology of the British Empire 49: 1–17

Chesley L C, Annitto J E 1947 Pregnancy in the patient with hypertensive disease. American Journal of Obstetrics and Gynecology 53: 372–381

Davey D A, MacGillivray I 1986 The classification and definition of the hypertensive disorders of pregnancy. Clinical and Experimental Hypertension (B) B5(1): 97

Davey D A, MacGillivray I 1988 The classification and definition of the hypertensive disorders of pregnancy. American Journal of Obstetrics and Gynecology 158: 892–898

Fisher K A, Luger A, Spargo B H et al 1981 Hypertension in pregnancy: clinical–pathological correlations and remote prognosis. Medicine 60: 267–276

National High Blood Pressure Education Program Working Group Report on High Blood Pressure in Pregnancy 1990 American Journal of Obstetrics and Gynecology 163: 1691–1712

Redman C W G, Jefferies M 1988 Revised definition of preeclampsia. Lancet 1: 809–812

WHO Study Group 1987 The hypertensive disorders of pregnancy. Technical Report Series no. 758. World Health Organization, Geneva, p 14–15

5.2 CLINICAL SYNDROMES IN HYPERTENSIVE DISORDERS OF PREGNANCY

When the blood pressure is found to be elevated in pregnancy the woman may have pregnancy induced hypertension which many would regard as synonymous with preeclampsia, or she may have underlying renal disease or essential hypertension. Underlying renal disease or essential hypertension is more likely if she is multiparous or has had hypertension in a previous pregnancy. Underlying renal disease is surprisingly common. Glomerulonephritis was demonstrated on renal biopsy in 38% of 123 women presenting with proteinuria in pregnancy (Kincaid-Smith & Fairley 1976). Fisher et al (1981) demonstrated glomerulonephritis in 22% of 176 consecutive patients presenting with hypertension in pregnancy.

Manifestations of preexisting hypertension or renal disease may be found in abnormal retinal vessels or cardiomegaly, or there may be a history of hypertension or renal disease prior to pregnancy.

Pregnancy induced hypertension or preeclampsia is more frequent in primipara and in those with a family history of preeclampsia (or eclampsia) in twin or multiple pregnancies and in association with a hydatidiform mole. Superimposed preeclampsia commonly occurs in women with underlying renal disease or diabetes and in those with essential hypertension.

Proteinuria without hypertension is much more likely to be a manifestation of underlying renal disease than of preeclampsia particularly if it occurs in the first or second trimester.

If one includes in the definition of preeclampsia or pregnancy induced hypertension a fall of blood pressure to normal levels within 3 months post partum, then in an individual case reclassification may be necessary in the postpartum period (Brown 1991).

In understanding gestational hypertension it is important to recognize the blood pressure changes which occur in normal women during pregnancy. Browne (1947) recommended that a blood pressure of 120/80 should be regarded as the upper limit of normal in early pregnancy. However, MacGillivray et al (1969), taking into consideration standardization of technique, found a lesser degree of fall in blood pressure in pregnancy than did Browne. The posture of the patient is important during pregnancy. Systolic blood pressure is 2–12 mmHg lower in the sitting position than with the patient recumbent (Fig. 5.2 –1).

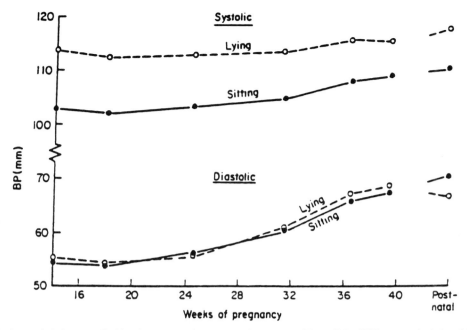

Fig. 5.2–1   Lying and sitting systolic blood pressures from 16 weeks to term. (From 'MacGillivray et al 1969, with permission.)

5.2.1 Gestational hypertension

Definitions of gestational hypertension are given in 5.1. Gestational hypertension is a broad category which includes patients with pregnancy induced hypertension, but no proteinuria, who do not therefore qualify for a diagnosis of preeclampsia. It includes a group of patients with late transient hypertension but excludes those with preeclampsia either primary or superimposed on preexisting hypertension or renal disease. Gestational hypertension also includes patients with known preexisting essential hypertension or renal disease, sometimes referred to as 'chronic hypertension'.

Opinions have varied about the relative importance of systolic and diastolic blood pressure levels. Browne (1947) used the systolic blood pressure level as an index of the severity of preeclampsia paying little attention to the diastolic blood pressure. Nelson (1955) stressed the importance of the diastolic blood pressure and this is now accepted for most definitions of preeclampsia which perhaps do not give sufficient weight to systolic blood pressure levels (see 5.1). Chesley & Annitto (1947) found a good correlation between systolic blood pressure and fetal outcome in 'chronic' hypertensive disease, and Tervila et al (1973) found

that the systolic blood pressure influenced the prognosis for the fetus in preeclampsia. Most obstetricians take both systolic and diastolic blood pressure into account and the importance of the maternal posture is well recognized.

Patients with preexisting hypertension often show a greater degree of decrease in blood pressure levels in early pregnancy than do normal women. Exaggerated decreases in blood pressure have been observed in some 40% of cases (Chesley & Annitto 1947, Browne 1947). In all pregnancies, the blood pressure tends to rise back to pre-pregnancy levels in the third trimester.

In patients with essential hypertension the risk of preeclampsia is increased three- to seven-fold and the greatest risk for the fetus is related to the development of superimposed preeclampsia. If superimposed preeclampsia does not occur, the outcome of pregnancy is stated to be the same as that of a normotensive pregnancy (Redman 1987a). In one large recent study, however, prematurity and small for gestational age (SGA) babies were twice as frequent in hypertensive pregnancies compared with normotensive pregnancies (Martikainen et al 1989). In this study, hypertension in pregnancy directly increased neonatal morbidity in preterm

SGA babies but this was related to preeclampsia. In full term babies, neonatal morbidity was not related to the severity of hypertension.

The reason for the higher rate of superimposed preeclampsia in women with essential hypertension is not known, but there are conspicuous hyperplastic changes in the uterine arteries in women with underlying hypertension (Robertson et al 1967) and these could predispose to failure of the normal trophoblast invasion of uterine arteries and hence lead to the development of the pathological lesions of preeclampsia in placental vessels and to consequent placental ischaemia.

Recurrence of hypertension in successive pregnancies is usually regarded as evidence of underlying renal disease or essential hypertension. One recent study has shown a significant association between HLA-DR4 antigens and the recurrence of hypertension in pregnancy. The biological significance of this observation is not clear (Simon et al 1988).

There is an association between age at first pregnancy and gestational hypertension. Antenatal hypertension is more frequent in primipara aged 40 or more (Brassil et al 1987).

Factors which predict the perinatal outcome in hypertensive pregnancies are proteinuria and early onset of hypertension (between 27 and 36 weeks). Both these risk factors are more frequent in women with no previous history of hypertension (Plouin et al 1986).

Continuing debate concerns the risk of hypertension developing in women as a late consequence of gestational hypertension. In a study of 446 cases of preeclampsia in which the blood pressure in early pregnancy was normal, the blood pressure 4 years after the pregnancy was higher than that of an unselected population of women of similar age (Gibson & Platt 1959). Subsequent studies have failed to confirm a higher risk of subsequent hypertension in women who have had preeclampsia. Adams & McGillivray (1961) found a higher average blood pressure reading after non proteinuric hypertension (perhaps reflecting underlying essential hypertension) than after proteinuric hypertension. In a more recent study (Svensson et al 1983) the best correlation with raised blood pressure after 7–12 years was a high systolic blood pressure in early pregnancy when the blood pressure is likely to reflect preexisting 'essential hypertension'. Lingeberg et al (1988) identified the gestational week at diagnosis as the best predictor of hypertension 5–6 years later, with subsequent hypertension occurring more frequently in those with an early onset in pregnancy.

In the above studies, the women who were hypertensive in early pregnancy are likely to be selecting out a group with preexisting hypertension or renal disease.

Chesley's classic studies in eclampsia (Chesley 1978) demonstrate that primipara who develop eclampsia have no increased risk of hypertension 33 years later (Fig. 5.2.1–1).

Severe hypertension in pregnancy may occur as a manifestation of preeclampsia but it may also occur in patients who do not have preeclampsia. We have frequently found an underlying cause such as reflux nephropathy in patients with severe hypertension in pregnancy.

Phaeochromocytoma may also present as severe hypertension in pregnancy and is associated with maternal death in 50–60% of cases not diagnosed before labour (Schenker & Grant 1982). Even if the diagnosis is made early in pregnancy, maternal death has occurred in up to 20% of cases. Fetal deaths occur in about half the cases, and it has been suggested that severe fetal complications may occur even with mild episodes of hypertension in women with phaeochromocytoma (Combs et al 1989).

In a recent series of 106 patients with severe hypertension in pregnancy (diastolic >120 mmHg on more than one occasion), fetal loss was as high as 20%, but the mothers all survived. Most patients in this series had proteinuric hypertension or preeclampsia.

5.2.2 Preeclampsia

Those who distinguish between preeclampsia and pregnancy induced hypertension do so on the basis of proteinuria as a feature of preeclampsia but not of pregnancy induced hypertension. Pregnancy induced hypertension without proteinuria is likely, however, to have similar underlying pathophysiological mechanisms (Brown 1991).

The prevalence of preeclampsia has probably not diminished (Redman 1987). Preeclampsia still occurs in some 10% of primiparous pregnancies.

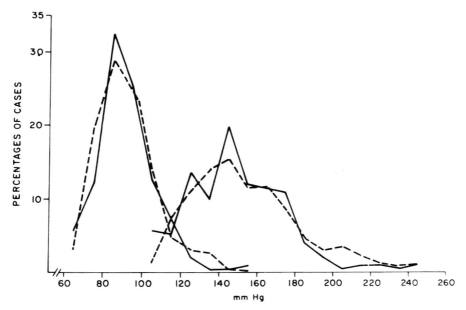

Fig. 5.2.1–1 The distributions of systolic and diastolic blood pressures in women who had eclampsia in the first pregnancy carried to viability (solid lines) compared with the distributions expected from the epidemiological study of Hamilton et al (1954) (broken lines). (From Chesley et al 1976, with permission.)

The underlying pathophysiological factors contributing to preeclampsia have been discussed earlier in Chapter 4.

It should be stressed in relation to the clinical syndrome of preeclampsia that, although this does not usually occur until the second half of pregnancy, two of the major underlying abnormalities — namely, increased vascular reactivity to angiotensin II and the failure of the process of trophoblast invasion and dilatation of placental vessels — are both well established by 14–16 weeks. The scene is thus set weeks or months before clinical manifestations appear. Where there is some underlying predisposing factor such as a twin pregnancy, renal disease or hydatidiform mole, preeclampsia has also been documented to occur in the first half of pregnancy. Fig. 5.2.2–1 shows characteristic morphological lesions of preeclampsia at 16 weeks' gestation in a patient without any obvious underlying predisposing factors. Eclampsia has also been documented in week 16 of pregnancy (Lindheimer et al 1974).

Patients with early onset preeclampsia very frequently show an underlying renal abnormality (Ihle et al 1987).

The early prediction of preeclampsia has special significance in relation to its treatment and prevention and is discussed under 5.3.

The clinical manifestations of preeclampsia are essentially those of hypertension and proteinuria. Oedema, if severe, should not be ignored because it may herald the onset of hypertension and proteinuria. The hypertension may be severe and the proteinuria is often in the nephrotic range.

A rise in blood pressure has particular significance in making the diagnosis and, whereas the WHO definition includes a rise in diastolic blood pressure of 15mm/Hg or more, Redman & Jefferies (1988) found that a rise in diastolic blood pressure of 25 mmHg better defined preeclampsia. They combined this very significant rise in diastolic blood pressure level with a first diastolic blood pressure below 90 mmHg and a maximum diastolic blood pressure above 90 mmHg and in doing so were able to exclude patients with 'chronic' hypertension.

Fallis & Langford (1963) observed a greater incidence of preeclampsia (toxaemia) in women whose blood pressures were in the high range of normal in the middle trimester. Hughes (1951)

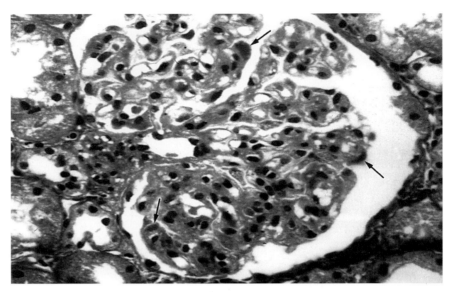

Fig. 5.2.2–1   Renal biopsy from a women who developed preeclampsia at 16 weeks' gestation, showing typical crescentic subendothelial deposits (arrows); clinical manifestations of severe hypertension and proteinuria disappeared rapidly after termination of pregnancy.

emphasized the importance of a rising diastolic blood pressure after 20 weeks' gestation as a warning sign of preeclampsia.

Oedema has been discarded as one of the three cardinal signs of preeclampsia because mild oedema is so common in normal pregnancy (Robertson 1971). Oedema is, however, a dramatic feature in some cases of preeclampsia and rapid weight gain of up to 10 kg may herald the onset of the other features of preeclampsia.

Only a minority of patients with preeclampsia develop proteinuria before they are hypertensive. Proteinuria was the first sign in only 3% of cases studied by Browne, whereas hypertension was the first sign in 75% (Browne 1933).

While the manifestations of preeclampsia persist, both the mother and the baby are at risk. There is no proven mechanism for reversing the signs of preeclampsia and, if spontaneous improvement does not occur with bed rest, or if the infant is not delivered, fetal death in utero may ensue. Once the baby is delivered, or fetal death occurs, rapid resolution of the features of preeclampsia in the mother follows.

More serious manifestations of preeclampsia appear in the so-called HELLP syndrome described by Weinstein in 1982. The syndrome is characterized by haemolysis, low platelets and elevation of liver enzymes. These manifestations probably all represent complications of intravascular coagulation and their clinical significance is that they are life threatening to the mother and demand urgent delivery. Pain in the right hypochondrium is a dangerous symptom in HELLP syndrome.

Thrombocytopenia can be life threatening in preeclampsia even when there is no liver involvement (Schwartz & Brenner 1983) and it may be confused with thrombotic thrombocytopenic purpura (Schwartz & Brenner 1978).

A rise in serum uric acid is probably the best biochemical test for monitoring the onset of preeclampsia (Chesley & Williams 1945). The degree of proteinuria increases with the severity of preeclampsia and the Tamm Horsfall protein level in the urine declines abruptly for reasons which are poorly understood. This change correlates with the severity of the disease (Nesselhut et al 1989).

The change in Tamm Horsfall protein may reflect a change in renal tubular function. Another alteration in tubular function is seen in the decreased fractional excretion of calcium which occurs in preeclampsia (Taufield et al 1987).

5.2.3 Eclampsia

Eclampsia, with its dramatic clinical manifestation of convulsions and its high mortality, was the major focus of interest until the beginning of this century when Schmorl (1901) noted that the typical pathological manifestations of eclampsia may be present in women who did not fit. Lever, as early as 1843, had pointed to proteinuria as a precursor of puerperal convulsions. Cook & Briggs (1903) wrote that an increase in blood pressure is an earlier and more reliable sign of impending convulsions than proteinuria. Eclampsia was more frequent before treatment was available to control the blood pressure (MacGillivray 1953), and eclampsia is now infrequently seen in modern obstetric services.

Improved antenatal care has obviously led to a decrease in the incidence and mortality of eclampsia in Western countries where eclampsia is now a rare complication of pregnancy. In Britain it occurs in less than 1 in 1000 deliveries (Redman 1988). In New Zealand the incidence fell from 3.2 per 1000 deliveries in 1928 to 0.8 per 1000 deliveries in 1958 (Corkill 1961). In New York, annual case mortality from eclampsia fell from 190 in 1920 to 3 in 1967 (Chesley 1978). The incidence of severe preeclampsia fell from 2.3% in 1965–1970 to 0.7% in 1970–1975; there were 28 cases of eclampsia in the first 5-year period (Hibbard & Rosen 1977) and only 12 in the second.

Eclampsia is seven to eight times as common in women who have had preeclampsia with proteinuria than in those without proteinuria. The cardinal clinical feature of eclampsia is the occurrence of convulsions. Other clinical features include proteinuria, impaired renal function and features of disseminated intravascular coagulation. The pathological basis for convulsions described by Schmorl (1901) was the presence of fibrin thrombi in arterioles and microscopic haemorrhages in the brain. Govan (1961) believed that fibrinoid necrosis in vascular walls was the primary lesion. Sheehan & Lynch (1973) described the pathological lesion of eclampsia as classically consisting of ring haemorrhages around a thrombosed precapillary. The lesions are distributed in the cortical gray matter and their distribution can be explained by cerebral autoregulation (Donaldson 1988).

Use of the newer imaging techniques of computed tomography and magnetic resonance imaging in 2 treated patients who recovered, showed disseminated transitory microvascular occlusions which resolved without residual detectable brain damage (Fredriksson et al 1989). In these two cases, neurological signs were preceded by a rapid increase in blood pressure and fall in platelet count. The period of thrombocytopenia corresponded with the maximum severity of lesions demonstrated by imaging techniques and, as the platelet count rose, the lesions resolved.

Before adequate antihypertensive treatment was available, the cause of death in eclampsia was most commonly cerebral (45%), often accompanied by cerebral haemorrhage; 30% of cases died from pulmonary oedema and only 5% from renal failure.

Convulsions can occur at relatively low blood pressure levels as eclampsia classically occurs in previously normotensive young women, and the lesions are likely to be caused by increased blood pressure and blood flow through a vascular bed not accustomed to these conditions (Donaldson 1988). In a few cases convulsions first develop 2–3 days post partum.

The treatment of eclampsia using hydralazine to lower the blood pressure and magnesium sulphate to control convulsions has dramatically reduced mortality. Pritchard & Pritchard (1975) reported 154 consecutive cases without any maternal mortality.

Eclampsia may be complicated by another potentially fatal condition, abruptio placentae (Lopez-Llera et al 1988). Maternal morality is high in such cases (21.7%), as is perinatal mortality (44.7%). Disseminated intravascular coagulation was recorded in 23% of cases and acute renal failure in 21% of cases complicated by abruptio placentae. There is some evidence that labour related eclampsia is becoming more common than antepartum eclampsia. Only 4 of 24 cases which occurred over 5 years in a Hong Kong hospital occurred ante partum, 10 of these developed in patients in whom hypertension first occurred during labour, none of whom had severe hypertension before the onset of convulsions (Lao et al 1987).

Although the official definition of eclampsia is often taken to be up to 24 h after delivery (Chesley

1978), cases of eclampsia have been recorded between 2 and 14 days after delivery (Brown et al 1987).

Chesley's classic studies on the remote prognosis of eclampsia (Chesley 1976) demonstrate unequivocally that there is no excess of observed over expected numbers of women with hypertension among primiparous eclamptic patients followed up many years later (Chesley 1978). Figure 5.2.1–1 shows the distribution of blood pressure in women who had eclampsia in the first pregnancy and the distribution in a normal population expected from an epidemiological survey — they are almost identical.

REFERENCES

Adams E M, MacGillivray I 1961 Long term effect of preeclampsia and blood pressure. Lancet 2: 1373–1375

Brassil M J, Turner M J, Egna D M et al 1987 Obstetric outcome in first-time mothers aged 40 years and over. European Journal of Obstetrics, Gynecology, and Reproductive Biology 25: 115–120

Brown M A 1991 Pregnancy-induced hypertension: pathogenesis and management. Australian and New Zealand Journal of Medicine 21: 257–273

Brown C E L, Cunningham F G, Pritchard J A 1987 Convulsions in hypertensive, proteinuric primiparas more than 24 hours after delivery: eclampsia or some other cause? Journal of Reproductive Medicine 32: 499–503

Browne F J 1933 The early signs of preeclamptic toxaemia, with special reference to the order of their appearance, and their inter-relation. Journal of Obstetrics and Gynaecology of the British Empire 40: 1160–1174

Browne F H 1947 Chronic hypertension in pregnancy. British Medical Journal 2:283–287

Chesley L C (ed) 1978 Hypertensive disorders in pregnancy. Appleton-Century-Crofts, New York, p 1–35, 53

Chesley L C, Annitto J E 1947 Pregnancy in the patient with hypertensive disease. American Journal of Obstetrics and Gynecology 53: 372–381

Chesley L C, Williams L O 1945 Renal glomerular and tubular function in relation to the hyperuricaemia of preeclampsia and eclampsia. American Journal of Obstetrics and Gynecology 50: 367–375

Chesley L C, Annitto J E, Cosgrove R A 1976 The remote prognosis of eclamptic women. Sixth periodic report. American Journal of Obstetrics and Gynecology 124: 446–459

Combs C A, Easterling T R, Schmucker B C et al 1989 Haemodynamic observations during paroxysmal hypertension in a pregnancy with pheochromocytoma. Obstetrics and Gynecology 74: 439–441

Conte G, Dal Canton A, Terribile M et al 1985 Exaggerated natriuresis in chronic hypertension in pregnancy (CHP). Kidney International 28: 233 (abstract)

Cook H W, Briggs J B 1903 Clinical observations on blood pressure. Johns Hopkins Hospital Report 11:451–534

Corkill T F 1961 Experience of toxaemia control in Australia and New Zealand. Pathologia et Microbiologia 24: 428–434

Donaldson J O 1988 Eclamptic hypertensive encephalopathy. Seminars in Nephrology 8: 230–233

Fallis N E, Langford H G 1963 Relation of second trimester blood pressure to toxaemia of pregnancy in the primigravid patient. American Journal of Obstetrics and Gynecology 87: 123–125

Fisher K A, Luger A, Spargo B H et al 1981 Hypertension in pregnancy: clinical-pathological correlations and remote prognosis. Medicine 60: 267–276

Fredriksson K, Lindvall O, Ingemarsson I et al 1989 Repeated cranial computed tomographic and magnetic resonance imaging scans in two cases of eclampsia. Stroke 20: 547–553

Gibson G B, Platt R 1959 Incidence of hypertension after pregnancy toxaemia. British Medical Journal 2: 159–162

Govan A D T 1961 The pathogenesis of eclamptic lesions. Pathologia et Microbiologia 24: 561–575

Hibbard B M, Rosen M 1977 The management of severe preeclampsia and eclampsia. British Journal of Anaesthesia 49: 3–9

Hughes T D 1951 The importance of the relativity of blood pressure and other signs in the prevention of eclampsia. Medical Journal of Australia 21: 871–874

Ihle B U, Long P, Oats J 1987 Early onset preeclampsia: recognition of underlying renal disease. British Medical Journal 294: 79–81

Kincaid-Smith P, Fairley K F 1976 The differential diagnosis between preeclamptic toxaemia and glomerulonephritis in patients with proteinuria in pregnancy. In: M D Lindheimer, A I Katz, F P Zuspan (eds) Hypertension in pregnancy. Wiley, New York, pp 157–167

Lao T T, Chin R K H, Leung B F H 1987 Labour-related eclampsia. European Journal of Obstetrics, Gynecology, and Reproductive Biology 26: 97–104

Lever J C W 1843 Cases of puerperal convulsions, with remarks. Guy's Hospital Reports Volume 1/2nd series 495–517

Lindheimer M D, Spargo B H, Katz A I 1974 Eclampsia during the 16th week of gestation. Journal of the American Medical Association 230: 1006–1008

Lingeberg S, Azelsson O, Jorner U et al 1988 A prospective controlled five-year follow-up study of primiparas with gestational hypertension. Acta Obstetricia et Gynaecologica Scandinavica 67: 605–609

Lopez-Llera M, de la Luz Espinosa M, Arratia C 1988 Eclampsia and placental abruption: basic patterns, management and morbidity. International Journal of Gynecology and Obstetrics 27: 335–342

MacGillivray I (ed) 1953 Preeclampsia and hypertensive disorders of pregnancy. WB Saunders, London

MacGillivray I, Rose G A, Rowe D 1969 Blood pressure survey in pregnancy. Clinical Science 37: 395–407

Martikainen A M, Jeompmem K M, Saarolpslo S V 1989 The effect of hypertension in pregnancy on foetal and neonatal condition. International Journal of Gynecology and Obstetrics 30: 213–220

National Institutes of Health Working group on High Blood Pressure in Pregnancy. N. I. H. Publication 91–3029 1991 U S Dept Health and Human Services

Nelson T R 1955 A clinical study of preeclampsia. Journal of

Obstetrics and Gynaecology of the British Commonwealth 62: 48–57

Nesselhut T, Rath W, Wever M H et al 1989 Veranderungen de Tam-Horsfall-Protennausscheidurg in Urin von Patientinnen mit Schwangerschaftshypertonie. Klinische Wochenschrift 67(suppl 17): 11–13

Plouin P F, Chatellier S, Breart S et al 1986 Factors predictive of perinatal outcome in pregnancies complicated by hypertension. European Journal of Obstetrics, Gynecology, and Reproductive Biology 23: 341–348

Pritchard J A, Pritchard S A 1975 Standardized treatment of 154 consecutive cases of eclampsia. American Journal of Obstetrics and Gynecology 123: 543–552

Redman C W 1987a Hypertension in pregnancy: a case discussion. Kidney International 32: 151–160

Redman C W G 1987b Therapy of non-preeclamptic hypertension in pregnancy. American Journal of Kidney Diseases 9: 324–327

Redman C W G 1988 Eclampsia still kills. British Medical Journal 296: 1209–1988

Redman C W, Jefferies M 1988 Revised definition of preeclampsia. Lancet 1: 809–812

Robertson E G 1971 The natural history of oedema during pregnancy. Journal of Obstetrics and Gynaecology of the British Commonwealth 78: 520–529

Robertson W B, Brosens I, Dixon G 1967 The pathological response of the vessels of the placental bed to hypertensive pregnancy. Journal of Pathology and Bacteriology 93: 581–592

Schenker J G, Granat M 1982 Phaeochromocytoma and pregnancy — an updated appraisal. Australian and New Zealand Journal of Obstetrics and Gynaecology 22: 1–10

Schmorl G 1901 Zur pathologischen Anatomie der Eklampsie. Verhandlungen der Deutschen Gesellschaft fur Gynekologie 9: 303–313

Schwartz M L, Brenner W E 1978 The obfuscation of eclampsia by thrombotic thrombocytopenic purpura. American Journal of Obstetrics and Gynecology 131: 18–24

Schwartz M L, Brenner W E 1983 Pregnancy-induced hypertension presenting with life-threatening thrombocytopenia. American Journal of Obstetrics and Gynecology 146: 756–757

Sheehan H L, Lynch J B (eds) 1973 Pathology of toxaemia of pregnancy. Churchill Livingstone, London

Simon P, Fauchet R, Pilorge M et al 1988 Association of H L A DR4 with the risk of recurrence of pregnancy hypertension. Kidney International 34 (suppl 25): S125–S128

Svensson A, Ahdersch B, Hansson L 1983 Prediction of later hypertension following a hypertensive pregnancy. Journal of Hypertension 1: 94–96

Taufield P A, Ales K L, Resnick L M et al 1987 Hypocalciuria in preeclampsia. New England Journal of Medicine 316: 715–718

Tervila L, Geocke C, Timonen S 1973 Estimation of gestosis of pregnancy (EPH-gestosis) Acta Obstetricia et Gynecologica Scandinavica 52: 235–243

Weinstein L 1982 Syndrome of haemolysis, elevated liver enzymes, and low platelet count: a severe consequence of hypertension in pregnancy. American Journal of Obstetrics and Gynecology 142: 159–167

5.3. THE EARLY DETECTION AND PREVENTION OF THE HYPERTENSIVE DISORDERS OF PREGNANCY

A better understanding of the underlying pathogenetic mechanisms in preeclampsia, together with the recognition that both the increased sensitivity to angiotensin II and the morphological placental vascular changes occur months before signs of preeclampsia appear, have stimulated considerable interest in the early detection or prediction of preeclampsia. Successful intervention in cases with a high risk of developing preeclampsia has intensified this interest (Beaufils et al 1985).

Beaufils et al (1985), on the basis of the significance of thrombotic lesions and evidence of intravascular coagulation in preeclampsia, treated 102 patients in a prospective random allocation trial of aspirin and dipyridamole given from 3 months' gestation. The patients were a high risk group with known hypertension, renal disease or previous complicated pregnancies. This study demonstrated a remarkable improvement in outcome in the treated group (Table 5.3–1).

Table 5.3–1 Outcome of pregnancy (from Beaufils 1985, with permission)

	Group A (n = 48)	Group B (n = 45)	P
Normal pregnancy	29	12	<0.005
Hypertension (isolated)	19	22	NS
Preeclampsia	0	6	<0.01
Fetal and neonatal loss	0	5	<0.02
Severe IUGR (live births)	0	4	<0.05

IUGR, intrauterine growth retardation.
Group A = treated group

Subsequent studies have confirmed Beaufils' observations (Wallenburg et al 1986, Schiff et al 1989, Benigni et al 1989) and if these results are combined they suggest that aspirin may be highly effective in preventing the development of preeclampsia and the serious fetal complications of intrauterine growth retardation and stillbirth (Table 5.3–2). Two large trials of aspirin reported at the 1992 meeting of the International Society for the Study of Hypertension in Pregnancy

Table 5.3–2 The effects of low dose aspirin therapy upon the development of pregnancy induced hypertension (PIH), intrauterine growth retardation (UGR) and stillbirth (from Brown 1991, with permission)
(Data compiled from Wallenburg et al 1986, Schiff et al 1989, Benigni et al 1989, Beaufils et al 1985)

	Aspirin ($n = 122$)	Placebo/control ($n = 115$)	P
PIH	6	32	<0.001
IUGR	12	31	<0.001
Stillbirth	1	7	<0.001

showed no benefit in the treated group in moderate or low risk pregnancies.

The method used to predict preeclampsia in the above studies was an invasive one, which is not always acceptable to hospital ethics committees at this time. It involves the angiotensin infusion test described by Gant et al (1973) in which angiotensin is infused until a rise in diastolic blood pressure of 20 mmHg is achieved.

If aspirin or any other preventive means is to be applied on a broad scale in the prevention of preeclampsia, which occurs in 10% of primipara, then a much less invasive test than the angiotensin infusion test is required to screen primipara and other high risk groups to determine which women are likely to develop preeclampsia.

The simplest method of all may be measuring the blood pressure. It is possible that preeclampsia can be predicted by blood pressure elevation early in pregnancy. Many studies have demonstrated higher second trimester blood pressures in women destined to develop hypertension in late pregnancy (Page & Christianson 1976, Phelan et al 1977, Oney & Kalhausen 1983, Gavette & Roberts 1987).

The major difficulty with these studies is the false negative rate, which means that only about 60% of patients who are destined to develop hypertension are likely to be detected in this way.

Continuous 24-h blood pressure recordings may improve the accuracy of blood pressure measurement in the prediction of preeclampsia. Preliminary results suggest that automated blood pressure recording improves the sensitivity, specificity and positive and negative predictive values of severe hypertension developing in late pregnancy (Mooney & Dalton 1990).

The roll-over test introduced in 1974 by Gant et al as a clinical test which may predict preeclampsia has not really proved to have a good predictive value in other hands (O'Brien 1990, Narvarez et al 1990).

A combination of the roll-over test and other tests such as the second trimester mean arterial blood pressure measurement improves the predictive value of pregnancy induced hypertension (Phelan et al 1977).

Because uterine ischaemia is thought to play an essential role in the development of preeclampsia, the recent interest in the doppler waveform recorded over the uterine artery in the prediction of preeclampsia is not surprising.

Controversy still exists as to the value of the uterine artery doppler waveform in the prediction of preeclampsia but evidence is growing which supports early observations that an abnormal uterine artery waveform is of value in predicting which patients will develop preeclampsia (Campbell et al 1986, Schulman et al 1987).

Numerous studies have been carried out in this new field and several suggest that this method has great promise as a predictive tool for preeclampsia (Campbell et al 1986, Schulman et al 1987, Steel et al 1988, Cameron et al 1988, Hanretty et al 1988, 1989, Kofinas et al 1988, 1990, Friedman et al 1989, Ducey et al 1989, Lowery et al 1990).

The position of the recording probe is important as is the placental site in relation to the site of the probe. Colour ultrasound is a great advantage in that it provides an accurate guide to the anatomy of the uterine vessels and the placental site.

Uterine artery doppler waveforms have been shown to correlate with morphological abnormalities in placental bed vessels (Steel et al 1988).

A large recent study shows a high sensitivity for prediction of hypertension associated with proteinuria and for prediction of intrauterine growth retardation (Table 5.3–3) (Steel et al 1990).

Uteroplacental doppler waveforms were used to identify a group of 148 women at high risk of developing pregnancy induced hypertension. These women were then allocated, at random, to aspirin 75 mg daily or placebo from 24 weeks of pregnancy. Aspirin treatment reduced the frequency of proteinuria hypertension and hypertension before 37 weeks' gestation. Low birth weight babies were also less frequent in the treated group (Table 5.3–4)

Table 5.3–3   Pregnancy outcome based on waveform analysis (from Steel et al 1990, with permission)

| | No. (%) of subjects | | | |
	Normal waveforms ($n = 896$)	Abnormal waveforms ($n = 118$)	95% CL (%)	P
Hypertension				
Alone	45 (5%)	29 (25%)	12–28	<0.001
With proteinuria	7 (0.8%)	12 (10%)	4–15	<0.001
With IUGR	0	15 (13%)	7–19	<0.001
Onset of hypertension				
<37 weeks	6 (0.7%)	18 (15%)	8–21	<0.001
<34 weeks	3 (0.4%)	13 (11%)	5–16	<0.001
Maximum blood pressure				
Systolic <160 mmHg	11 (1%)	13 (11%)	4–16	<0.001
Diastolic <110 mmHg	8 (0.9%)	13 (11%)	4–16	<0.001
Hypotensive agents				
Oral only	2 (0.2%)	3 (2.5%)	−1–5	0.007
Intravenous	1 (0.1%)	6 (5.0%)	1–9	<0.001
Gestation at onset of labour				
<37 weeks	1 (0.1%)	21 (18%)	10–25	<0.001
<34 weeks	1 (0.1%)	9 (8%)	3–12	<0.001
IUGR				
Symmetrical	18 (2%)	4 (3%)	−2–5	NS
Asymmetrical	28 (3%)	23 (20%)	9–24	<0.001
Birthweight				
<5th centile	28 (3%)	21 (18%)	8–22	<0.001
10th centile	65 (7%)	32 (27%)	12–28	<0.001
Perinatal deaths				
Stillbirths	8 (0.9%)	3 (3%)	−1–5	NS
Neonatal deaths	2 (0.2%)	2 (2%)	−1–4	NS
Total	10 (1%)	5 (4%)	0–7	0.03

IUGR, intrauterine growth retardation; NS, not significant;
95% CL, 95% confidence limits for difference in proportions.

Table 5.3–4   Pregnancy outcome (from McPharland et al 1990, with permission)

	Placebo group	Aspirin group	95% CL (%)	p
No. (%) with				
Pregnancy induced hypertension	13 (25%)	6 (13%)	−3–28	NS
Proteinuric hypertension	10 (19%)	1 (2%)	6–29	<0.02
Onset of hypertension before week 37	9 (17%)	0	7–27	<0.01
Mean (SD)				
Gestation at delivery (weeks)	38.7 (3.9)	39.5 (2.1)	–	NS
Birthweight (g)	2954 (852)	3068 (555)	–	NS
No. (%) of infants				
<2500 g	13 (25%)	7 (15%)	−5–25	NS
<1500 g	4 (8%)	0	0–15	NS
Below 5th centile	7 (14%)	7 (14%)	–	NS
Mean (SD) blood loss at delivery (ml)	358 (228)	289 (188)	–	NS
Perinatal deaths	3	1	–	NS

95% CL, 95% confidence limits for difference in proportions; NS, not significant.

(McPharland et al 1990). Other similar studies are being carried out. Calcium supplementation of the diet has recently been reported to reduce the risk of preeclampsia (Belizan et al 1991). The rate of hypertension was 9.8% in the treated group and 14.8% in the placebo group ($P<0.001$).

Page (1948) first proposed using heparin to treat preeclampsia. Heparin and dipyridamole have been used in high risk pregnancies (Bonnar et al 1975, 1976) with apparent benefit. This is discussed in 5.4 and 6.13. This combination has also been shown to be of benefit in patients with renal disease as discussed in 5.4 and 6.13.

REFERENCES

Beaufils M, Uzan S, Donslmoni R et al 1985 Prevention of preeclampsia by early antiplatelet therapy. Lancet 1: 840–842

Belizan J M, Villar J, Gonzailez L et al 1991 Calcium supplementation to prevent hypertensive disorders of pregnancy. New England Journal of Medicine 325: 1399–1405

Benigni A, Gregorini G, Frusca T et al 1989 Effect of low-dose aspirin on foetal and maternal generation of thromboxane by platelets in women at risk for pregnancy-induced hypertension. New England Journal of Medicine 321: 357–362

Bonnar J, Redman C W G, Sheppard B L 1975 Treatment of fetal growth retardation in utero with heparin and dipyridamole. European Journal of Obstetrics, Gynecology, and Reproductive Biology 5: 123–134

Bonnar J, Redman C W G, Denson K W 1976 The role of coagulation and fibrinolysis in preeclampsia. In: M D Lindheimer, A L Katz, F P Zuspan (eds) Hypertension in pregnancy. Wiley, New York, p 85

Brown M A 1991 Pregnancy-induced hypertension: pathogenesis and management. Australian and New Zealand Journal of Medicine 21: 257–273

Cameron A D, Nicholson SF, Nimrod C A et al 1988 Doppler waveforms in the foetal aorta and umbilical artery in patients with hypertension in pregnancy. American Journal of Obstetrics and Gynecology 158: 339–345

Campbell S, Pearce J M F, Hackett G et al 1986 Qualitative assessment of uteroplacental blood flow: early screening test for high-risk pregnancies. Obstetrics and Gynecology 68:649–653

Ducey J 1989 Velocity waveforms in hypertensive disease. Clinical Obstetrics and Gynecology 32: 679–686

Ducey J, Schulman H, Farmakides G et al 1987 A classification of hypertension in pregnancy based on Doppler velocimetry. American Journal of Obstetrics and Gynecology 157: 680–685

Gant N F, Daley G L, Chand S et al 1973 A study of angiotensin II pressor response throughout primigravid pregnancy. Journal of Clinical Investigation 52: 2682–2689

Freidman D M, Ehrlich P, Hoskins I A 1989 Umbilical artery Doppler blood velocity waveforms in normal and abnormal gestation. Journal of Ultrasound in Medicine 8: 375–380

Gant N F, Chand S, Worley R J, et al 1974 A clinical test

useful for predicting the development of acute hypertension in pregnancy. American Journal of Obstetrics and Gynecology 20: 1–7

Gavette L, Roberts J 1987 Use of mean arterial pressure (MAP–2) to predict pregnancy-induced hypertension in adolescents. Journal of Nurse-Midwifery 32: 357–364

Hanretty K P, Whittle M J, Rubin P C 1988 Doppler uteroplacental waveforms in pregnancy-induced hypertension: a re-appraisal. Lancet 1: 850–852

Hanretty K P, Primrose M H, Neilson J P et al 1989 Pregnancy screening by Doppler uteroplacental and umbilical artery waveforms. British Journal of Obstetrics and Gynaecology 96: 1163–1167

Kofinas A D, Penry M, Greiss F C et al 1988 American Journal of Obstetrics and Gynecology 159: 1504–1504

Kofinas A D, Penry M, Nelson L H et al 1990 Uterine and umbilical artery flow velocity waveform analysis in pregnancies complicated by chronic hypertension or preeclampsia. Southern Medical Journal 83: 150–155

Lowery CL, Henson BV, Wan J et al 1990 A comparison between umbilical artery velocimetry and standard antepartum surveillance in hospitalized high-risk patients. American Journal of Obstetrics and Gynecology 162: 710–714

McPharland P, Pearce J M, Champerlain G V P 1990 Doppler ultrasound and aspirin in recognition and prevention of pregnancy-induced hypertension. Lancet 355: 1552–1555

Mooney P, Dalton K J 1990 An 'admission challenge test' to predict severe hypertension in pregnancy? European Journal of Obstetrics, Gynecology, and Reproductive Biology 35: 41–49

Narvarez M, Weigel M M, Felix C et al 1990 The clinical utility of the roll-over test in predicting pregnancy-induced hypertension in a high-risk Andean population. International Journal of Gynecology and Obstetrics 31: 9–14

O'Brien W F 1990 Predicting preeclampsia. Obstetrics and Gynecology 75: 445–452

Oney T, Kaulhausen H 1983 The value of the mean arterial blood pressure in the second trimester (MAP–2 value) as a predictor of pregnancy-induced hypertension and preeclampsia: a preliminary report. Clinical and Experimental Hypertension Part B Hypertension in Pregnancy: 211–216

Page E W 1948 Heparin and toxaemia of pregnancy. Obstetrical and Gynecological Survey 3: 615

Page E W, Christianson R 1976 The impact of mean arterial blood pressure in the middle trimester upon the outcome of pregnancy. American Journal of Obstetrics and Gynecology 125: 740–745

Phelan J P, Everidge G J, Wilder T L et al 1977 Is the supine pressor test an adequate means of predicting acute hypertension in pregnancy? American Journal of Obstetrics and Gynecology 129: 397–400

Schiff E, Peleg E, Goldenberg M et al 1989 The use of aspirin to prevent pregnancy-induced hypertension and lower the ratio of thromboxane A_2 to prostacyclin in relatively high risk pregnancies. New England Journal of Medicine 321: 351–356

Schulman H, Ducey J, Farmakides G et al 1987 Uterine artery Doppler velocimetry: the significance of divergent systolic/diastolic ratios. American Journal of Obstetrics and Gynecology 157:1539–1542

Steel SA, Pearce JM, Chamberlain GV 1988 Doppler

ultrasound of the uteroplacental circulation as a screening test for severe preeclampsia with intra-uterine growth retardation. European Journal of Obstetrics, Gynecology, and Reproductive Biology 28:279–287

Steel S A, Pearce J M, Chamberlain G V P 1990 Early Doppler ultrasound screening in prediction of hypertensive disorders of pregnancy. Lancet 335: 1548–1551

Wallenburg H C S, Dekker G A, Makovitz J W et al 1986 Low-dose aspirin prevents pregnancy-induced hypertension and preeclampsia in angiotensin-sensitive primigravidae. Lancet 1: 1–3

5.4 MANAGEMENT AND DRUG TREATMENT OF HYPERTENSIVE DISORDERS OF PREGNANCY

In discussing management of hypertension during pregnancy, a number of aspects need to be considered.

Control of the blood pressure in a woman with preeclampsia is considered separately from control of the blood pressure in a patient already on treatment prior to pregnancy for what is usually called 'chronic' hypertension.

The influence of individual antihypertensive drugs on placental blood flow has probably not received sufficient attention. Potential teratogenic and other adverse effects of drugs on the fetus must also be considered in treating hypertension in pregnancy.

5.4.1 Sodium intake in pregnancy

Sodium restriction was widely practised in pregnancy in the early days of antenatal care to control the frequent oedema seen in pregnant women.

Oedema is a characteristic feature of preeclampsia in spite of a low plasma volume (Freis & Kenny 1948) and abnormal sodium retention occurs in preeclampsia (Chesley 1978). It is not surprising, therefore, that salt restriction has been used in an attempt to prevent or control the oedema of preeclampsia (De Snoo 1937).

Robinson (1958), in a controlled trial of the effect of salt restriction in 2019 pregnant women, found that the incidence of hypertension oedema and proteinuria was higher in women instructed to reduce their salt intake than in those on a normal or high salt intake.

Pregnant women select a diet high in sodium (Kalousek et al 1969). Sarles et al (1968) found

that they had to give pregnant women 100 mEq of sodium daily to maintain sodium balance.

Few would advise sodium restriction for the prevention or treatment of preeclampsia at the present time.

5.4.2 Diuretics

In the same way as sodium restriction has been practised in an attempt to control or prevent the manifestation of preeclampsia, diuretics were widely used in the early 1960s in the hope that, in preventing the hypertension and oedema, they might prevent preeclampsia. There were a few isolated reports of intrauterine death in women treated with chlorothiazide to control oedema (Watt & Philip 1960) and diuretics have been used little in pregnancy hypertension since that time.

A meta-analysis of randomized trials of the value of diuretics in the prevention of preeclampsia, conducted over 20 years, included 7000 patients. Even when oedema was not included as evidence of preeclampsia, there was overwhelming evidence in this analysis that the signs of preeclampsia could be prevented by diuretics (Collins et al 1985). The incidence of stillbirths was reduced by a third in the treated group; however, this was not statistically significant. In order to demonstrate a significant difference in stillbirths, Collins et al (1985) concluded that tens of thousands of pregnancies may need to be studied in controlled trials. This meta-analysis does, however, demonstrate that diuretics are not harmful when used in pregnancy. They are most commonly used at the present time in women who are being treated with diuretics for hypertension prior to pregnancy and who continue to take them during pregnancy.

5.4.3 Lowering the blood pressure in patients with preeclampsia

Although bed rest may sometimes improve the clinical manifestations in patients with preeclampsia, in general it is desirable to deliver the baby as soon as possible.

Control of the blood pressure using antihypertensive drugs may be necessary, particularly when the blood pressure is very high and eclampsia or intracerebral haemorrhage may occur (Redman 1988).

Although very severe hypertension may occur in pregnancy in the context of so-called 'chronic' hypertension or underlying disease such as renal artery stenosis or phaeochromocytoma, it is most commonly seen in preeclampsia.

The blood pressure can be controlled by a wide range of drugs but rapid reduction is probably best achieved by vasodilators such as intravenous hydralazine (Mabie et al 1987). The powerful vasodilator diazoxide (Barr & Gallery 1981) is little used now that alternative methods are available. Oral (Walters & Redman 1984) or sublingual (Lindow et al 1988) nifedipine has also proved effective for rapid blood pressure reduction. In addition to vasodilators, the combined α- and β-adrenergic blocking agent, labetalol, has been used intravenously (Mabie et al 1987). Most drugs used to lower the blood pressure rapidly will reduce uterine blood flow and may cause fetal death (Nylund & Lunell 1988). Uterine artery doppler waveform monitoring may be useful for monitoring fetal blood supply (Hanretty et al 1989).

Preeclampsia is the major cause of fetal loss, and to modify its course significantly treatment would need to be started early in pregnancy, probably about 12–14 weeks, to modify both the placental vascular lesions of preeclampsia and the increased vascular reactivity. No large scale trial has been done commencing treatment at an early stage in pregnancy; indeed this could only be done if an accurate method of prediciting preeclampsia became available.

5.4.4 Lowering the blood pressure in patients with so-called 'chronic' hypertension and secondary hypertension

Renal disease is by far the commonest cause of secondary hypertension in pregnancy. In patients with renal disease, the management is similar to that in patients with essential hypertension discussed below.

Tumours of the adrenal gland rarely cause hypertension in pregnancy and of these the one which causes the most concern is phaeo-chromocytoma because of the high risk of death of the mother and fetus (Fudge et al 1980,

Schenker & Chowers 1971). Management by α- and β-adrenergic blocking drugs and where possible definitive surgery during pregnancy is recommended (Fudge et al 1980).

Primary aldosteronism (Hammond et al 1982) is rare and usually presents as hypertension associated with hypokalaemia and metabolic alkalosis. Surgery is not indicated during pregnancy which progresses satisfactorily provided the hypokalaemia is corrected. Surgical cure of hypertension is desirable if further pregnancies are planned.

Cushing's syndrome is also rare; Gormley et al (1982) reviewed 34 pregnancies. The incidence of stillbirth and spontaneous abortion is high. Symptoms of Cushing's disease may recede during pregnancy and surgery where indicated is usually carried out after pregnancy.

The uterine artery branches in women with secondary or chronic hypertension in pregnancy show marked intimal hyperplasia, which develops before 20 weeks. Almost all treatment trials have been carried out after 20 weeks' gestation and therefore it is not known whether treatment can prevent these lesions.

None of the controlled trials of antihypertensive drug treatment in pregnancy show clear cut benefit in the treated group. If, however, the trials are pooled and subjected to so-called meta-analysis, benefit does merge with a relative risk of fetal mortality of 0.37 in the treated group (Fletcher & Bulpitt 1988). A large trial would be needed to confirm the benefit of treatment suggested by this meta-analysis.

Similar problems exist for a comparison of the different antihypertensive drugs used in pregnancy. Three large trials have been carried out. Two compared methyldopa with oxprenolol (Fidler et al 1983, Gallery et al 1979). Both were open studies and neither showed any difference in fetal mortality. In a subsequent paper Gallery et al (1985) found a higher birth weight for gestational age in the oxprenolol treated group. The fact that this difference was greatest in babies of mothers treated for the shortest time has led to some confusion about the findings.

The effect of atenolol on fetal growth appears to be different from that claimed above for oxprenolol (Rubin et al 1983). Although the babies were smaller in the atenolol group, less proteinuria and less neonatal respiratory disease was observed in the treated group.

The view most commonly expressed at the present time is that treatment of mild to moderate hypertension in pregnancy does not prevent the development of superimposed preeclampsia (Redman 1991).

The trials which have been done and their outcome are summarized in Table 5.4.4–1.

Severe hypertension in pregnancy clearly needs to be treated because of the maternal risk.

The outcome for the baby is very poor in severe hypertension (Derham et al 1989). In a series of 106 patients in whom management was optimized, only 80% of babies survived. The gestational age was the major determinant of a healthy baby; 1 mother developed eclampsia, 1 pulmonary oedema and 1 acute renal failure.

Few controlled trials have been carried out in severe hypertension. Redman (1991) and Fletcher & Bulpitt (1988), in an interim analysis of 74 patients with a blood pressure above 170/110 allocated at random to labetalol 400 mg daily or methyldopa 800 mg daily, reported no real difference in results. Proteinuria developed in 1 of 25 treated with methyldopa and 3 of 22 treated with labetolol, and two deaths occurred in the labetolol group but none in the methyldopa group. The authors concluded that labetolol was effective but not superior to methyldopa.

While α- and β-adrenergic receptor antagonists have been widely used and these, together with methyldopa and labetalol, are regarded as safe in pregnancy, clearly some of the newer drugs are contraindicated. Converting enzyme inhibitors have caused fetal death in several animal species and acute renal failure in the newborn (Schubiger et al 1988, Anonymous 1989).

The value of calcium channel blocking agents is still being evaluated.

Slow release nifedipine has been evaluated in a small study and shown no serious side-effects (Constantine et al 1987); and a single dose nifedipine study suggests that calcium channel blockers may have a special role in severe hypertension in pregnancy (Horn et al 1990).

A marked fall in blood pressure accompanied nifedipine treatment in 2 women with preeclampsia who had failed to respond to methyldopa and magnesium sulphate (Waisman et al 1988).

Table 5.4.4–1 Controlled trials of antihypertensive treatment in pregnancy (modified from Redman 1991, with permission)

Reference	No. of subjects	Entry time (week)	Diagnosis	Active treatment (control group)	Effects of treatment*
Leather et al 1968	100	NR	HT	Methyldopa ± diuretic (none)	None
Redman et al 1976	207	21–22	CHT	Methyldopa (none)	Fewer perinatal and midtrimester losses
Weitz et al 1987	25	NR	CHT	Methyldopa (placebo#)	None
Rubin et al 1983	86	34	HT	Atenolol (placebo#)	Less proteinuria, fewer hospital admissions, more neonatal bradycardia
Butters et al 1990	29	16	CHT	Atenolol (placebo#)	Intrauterine growth retardation
Pickles et al 1989	152	34	PIH	Labetolol (placebo#)	None
Sibai et al 1987	100	33	PE	Labetolol (bed rest)	Intrauterine growth retardation
Wichman et al 1984	52	33	HT	Metoprolol (placebo#)	Fetal bradycardia, lower umbilical venous lactate
Plouin et al	155	28	PIH	Oxprenolol ± hydralazine (placebo#)	Fewer caesarian sections, less prolonged neonatal care
Gallery et al 1985	183	29–30	HT	Oxprenolol (methyldopa)	Better intrauterine growth
Fidler et al 1983	100	30–31	HT	Oxprenolol (methyldopa)	None
Thorley 1984	60	NR	HT	Atenolol (methyldopa)	Lower placental weights
Redman 1982	72	31	HT	Labetolol (methyldopa)	None
Mabie et al 1987	60		PHT	Labetolol (hydralazine)	None
Barton et al 1990	31		PPHT	Nifedipine (placebo#)	More urine output in first 24 h after delivery

NR, not recorded; PIH, pregnancy induced hypertension; CHT, chronic hypertension; HT, hypertension unqualified; PPHT, postpartum hypertension; PHT, peripartum hypertension; PE, preeclampsia.
*Excluding lower blood pressures and statistically non-significant effects.
#Double-blind allocation of treatment.

5.4.5 Heparin and dipyridamole

The prominence of fibrin in placental vessels has led two groups, Bonnar's (Bonnar et al 1975) and our own (Whitworth & Fairley 1973, Fairley et al 1976), to use dipyridamole and heparin in the treatment of preeclampsia.

Bonnar et al (1975) reported on the use of heparin and dipyridamole in 16 women with strong evidence of compromised fetoplacental function; 14 of the 16 women were able to continue the pregnancy for periods of weeks and achieved live infants in all 14. In a similar study in Melbourne, 9 patients were treated with heparin and dipyridamole and improvement permitted continuation of pregnancy, resulting in 6 living babies. The use of heparin and dipyridamole in both studies seemed to permit continuation of pregnancy to a stage where the baby was viable. This is less important now than it was when the above studies were carried out because neonatal paediatric care has improved significantly in small premature infants. Reversal of the glomerular lesion of preeclampsia was achieved on renal biopsy (Fairley et al 1976). We have conducted controlled trials of heparin and dipyridamole in high risk pregnancies in patients with renal disease; this is discussed in 6.13.

In any woman with hypertension in pregnancy, persistence of the hypertension and/or proteinuria 3 months after pregnancy warrants investigation for an underlying cause because this excludes preeclampsia as the cause of hypertension and proteinuria. A high percentage of women with hypertension or proteinuria in pregnancy have underlying renal disease (Kincaid-Smith & Fairley 1976, Fisher et al 1981). Glomerulonephritis and reflux nephropathy are among the most frequent lesions diagnosed in such patients, but other underlying diseases such as renal artery stenosis, aldosterone secreting tumour and phaeochromocytoma may also be present as the cause of hypertension in pregnancy and require specific management.

REFERENCES

Anonymous 1989 Are A C E inhibitors safe in pregnancy? Lancet 2: 482–483

Barr PA, Gallery E D M 1981 Effect of diazoxide on the antepartum cardiotocograph in severe pregnancy associated hypertension. Australian and New Zealand Journal of Obstetrics and Gynaecology 21: 11–15

Barton J R, Hiett A K, Conover W B 1990 The use if nifedipine during the postpartum period in patients with severe preeclampsia. American Journal of Obstetrics and Gynecology 162: 788–792

Bonnar J, Redman C W G, Sheppard B L 1975 Treatment of fetal growth retardation in utero with heparin and dipyridamole. European Journal of Obstetrics, Gynecology, and Reproductive Biology 5: 123–134

Butters L, Kennedy S, Rubin P C 1990 Atenolol in the mangement of essential hypertension during pregnancy. British Medical Journal 301: 587–589

Chesley L A (ed) 1978 Hypertension disorders in pregnancy. Appleton-Century-Crofts, New York, pp 225

Collins R, Yusuf S, Peto R 1985 Overview of randomised trials of diuretics in pregnancy. British Medical Journal 290: 17–23

Constantine G, Beevers D G, Reynolds A L et al 1987 Nifedipine as a second line antihypertensive drug in pregnancy. British Journal of Obstetrics and Gynecology 94: 1136–1142

Derham R J, Hawkins D F, De Vries L S et al 1989 Outcome of pregnancies complicated by severe hypertension and delivered before 34 weeks; stepwise logistic regression analysis of prognostic factors. British Journal of Obstetrics and Gynaecology 96: 1173–1181

De Snoo K 1937 The prevention of eclampsia. American Journal of Obstetrics and Gynecology 34: 911–926

Fairley K F, Adey F D, Ross I C et al 1976 Heparin treatment in severe preeclampsia and glomerulonephritis in pregnancy. In: M D Lindheimer, A I Katz, F P Zuspan (eds) Hypertension in pregnancy. Wiley, New York, pp 103–112

Fidler J, Smith V, Fayers P et al 1983 Randomised controlled comparative study of methyl dopa and oxprenolol for the treatment of hypertension in pregnancy. British Medical Journal 286: 1927–1930

Fisher K A, Luger A, Spargo B H et al 1981 Hypertension in pregnancy: clinical–pathology correlations and remote prognosis. Medicine 60: 267–276

Fletcher A E, Bulpitt C J 1988 A review of clinical trials in pregnancy hypertension. In: P C Rubin (ed) Handbook of hypertension. Elsevier, Amsterdam, vol 10: 186–201

Freis E D, Kenny J F 1948 Plasma volume, total circulating protein, and 'available fluid' abnormalities in preeclampsia and eclampsia. Journal of Clinical Investigation 27: 283–289

Fudge T L, McKinnon W M P, Geary W L 1980 Current surgical management of pheochromocytoma during pregnancy. Archives of Surgery 115: 1224–1225

Gallery E D M, Saunders D M, Hunyor S N et al 1979 Randomised comparison of methyldopa and oxprenolol for treatment of hypertension in pregnancy. British Medical Journal 1: 1591–1594

Gallery E D M, Ross M R, Gyory A Z 1985 Antihypertensive treatment in pregnancy: analysis of different responses to oxprenolol and methyldopa. British Medical Journal 291: 563–566

Gormley M J J, Hadden D R, Kennedy T L et al 1982 Cushing's syndrome in pregnancy — treatment with metyrapone. Clinical Endocrinology 16: 282–293

Hammond T G, Buchanan J D, Scoggins B A et al 1982 Primary hyperaldosteronism in pregnancy. Australian and

New Zealand Journal of Medicine 12: 537–539

Hanretty K P, Whittle M J, Howie C A et al 1989 Effect of nifedipine on doppler flow velocity waveforms in severe preeclampsia. British Medical Journal 299: 1205–1205

Horn E H, Filshie M, Kerslake R W et al 1990 Widespread cerebral ischaemia treated with nimodipine in a patient with eclampsia. British Medical Journal 301: 794

Kalousek G, Hlavacek C, Nedoss B et al 1969 Circadian rhythms of creatinine and electrolyte excretion in healthy pregnant women. American Journal of Obstetrics and Gynecology 103: 856–867

Kincaid-Smith P, Fairley K F 1976 The differential diagnosis between preeclamptic toxaemia and glomerulonephritis in patients with proteinuria in pregnancy In: M D Lindheimer, AI Katz, F P Zuzpan (ed) Hypertension in pregnancy. Wiley, New York, pp 157–167

Leather H M, Humphreys D M, Baker P et al 1968 A controlled trial of hypotensive agents in hypertension in pregnancy. Lancet 2: 488–490

Lindow S W, Davies N, Davey D A et al 1988 The effect of sublingual nifedipine on uteroplacental blood flow in hypertensive pregnancy. British Journal of Obstetrics and Gynaecology 95: 1276–1281

Mabie W C, Gonzaler A R, Sibai B M et al 1987 A comparative trial of labetalol and hydralazine in the acute management of severe hypertension complicating pregnancy. Obstetrics and Gynecology 70: 328–333

Nylund L, Lunell N–O 1988 Dihydralazine and the uteroplacental blood flow. American Journal of Obstetrics and Gynecology 158: 440–441

Pickles C J, Symonds E M, Broughton Pipkin F 1989 The fatal outcome in a randomized double-blind controlled trial of labetalol versus placebo in pregnancy-induced hypertension. British Journal of Obstetrics and Gynaecology 96:38–43

Redman C W G 1982 A controlled trial of the treatment of hypertension in pregnancy: labetalol compared with methyldopa. In: A Riley, E M Symonds (eds) Investigation of labetalol in the management of hypertension in pregnancy. International Congress Series 591, Excerpta Medica, Amsterdam, p 101–110

Redman C W G 1988 Eclampsia still kills. British Medical Journal 296: 1209–1210

Redman C W G 1991 Controlled trials of antihypertensive drugs in pregnancy. American Journal of Kidney Diseases 17: 149–153

Redman C W G, Belilin L J, Bonnar J et al 1976 Fetal

outcome in trial of antihypertensive treatment in pregnancy. Lancet 2:753–756

Robinson M 1958 Salt in pregnancy. Lancet 1: 178–181

Rubin P C, Butters L, Clark D M et al 1983 Placebo-controlled trial of atenolol in treatment of pregnancy-associated hypertension. Lancet 2: 431–434

Sarles H E, Hill S S, LeBlanc A L et al 1968 Sodium excretion patterns during and following intravenous sodium chloride loads in normal and hypertensive pregnancies. American Journal of Obstetrics and Gynecology 102: 1–7

Schenker J G, Chowers I 1971 Pheochromocytoma and pregnancy. Review of 89 cases. Obstetrical and Gynecological Survey 26: 739–747

Schubiger G, Flury G, Nassberger J 1988 Enalapril for pregnancy-induced hypertension: acute renal failure in a neonate. Annals of Internal Medicine 108: 215–216

Sibai B M, Gonzalez A R, Mabie W C et al 1987 A comparison of labetalol plus hospitalization versus hospitalization alone in the management of preeclampsia remote from term. Obstetrics and Gynecology 70: 323–327

Thorley K J 1984 Randomised trial of atenolol and methyldopa in pregnancy related hypertension. Clinical and Experimental Hypertension Part B Hypertension in Pregnancy 3: 168

Waisman G D, Mayorga L M, Camera M I et al 1988 Magnesium plus nifedipine: potentiation of hypotensive effect in preeclampsia? American Journal of Obstetrics and Gynecology 159: 308–109

Walters B N J, Redman C W G 1984 Treatment of severe pregnancy-associated hypertension with the calcium antagonist nifedipine. British Journal of Obstetrics and Gynaecology 91: 330–336

Watt J D, Philip E E 1960 Oral diuretics in pregnancy toxaemia. British Medical Journal 1: 1807

Weitz C, Khouzami V, Maxwell K et al 1987 Treatment of hypertension in pregnancy with methyldopa: a randomised double blind study. International Journal of Gynecology and Obstetrics 25: 35–40

Whichman K, Ryden G, Karlberg B E 1984 A placebo controlled trial of metoprolol in the treatment of hypertension in pregnancy. Scandinavian Journal of Clinical and Laboratory Investigation 44(suppl): 90–95

Whitworth J A, Fairley K F 1973 Heparin in the treatment of preeclamptic toxaemia In: P Kincaid-Smith, T H Mathew, E L Becker (eds) Glomerulonephritis. Wiley, New York p 1027

6. Renal and urinary tract disorders in pregnancy

6.1 BACTERIURIA AND URINARY TRACT INFECTION

Rayer (1839–1841) first drew attention to pyelonephritis occurring in pregnancy, and in 1892 Reblaub described 5 cases of urinary tract infection in pregnancy and implicated compression of the ureters by the uterus as a causative factor. Early this century, Albeck (1907) reported the presence of *Escherichia coli* in pure culture in the urine in 80% of pregnant women with bacteriuria.

Dodds (1931) was the first to study a consecutive series of pregnant women for the presence of bacteriuria and she found coliform bacteria in the urine in 7.6% of these women and other organisms in the urine in 3.6% of 406 antenatal patients.

Urinary tract infection can be present in three different clinical contexts in pregnancy: namely, as asymptomatic bacteriuria, symptomatic acute cystitis and symptomatic acute pyelonephritis.

6.1.1 Asymptomatic bacteriuria

Asymptomatic bacteriuria, although recognized as a common accompaniment of pregnancy, received little attention in early obstetric text books except as a confounding factor in the diagnosis of acute pyelonephritis. It was recognized that heavy pyuria accompanied acute pyelonephritis and, whereas the presence of bacteriuria in the urine was not a useful diagnostic criterion because of its frequency in women without symptoms, the presence of heavy pyuria was claimed to support a diagnosis of acute pyelonephritis. The common method of microscopy was to place a uncentrifuged drop of urine on a slide and the presence of pus cells indicated heavy pyuria; indeed, 1 pus cell per high powered field using this method is equivalent to approximately 25 000 leucocytes per ml of urine — well above the upper limit of normal of 2000 per ml.

After Dodds' (1931) careful studies, the literature contained very little about bacteriuria until Kass's important observation almost 30 years later that asymptomatic bacteriuria predisposes to acute pyelonephritis (Kass 1959).

Kass (1955) had earlier undertaken a systematic analysis of bacterial counts in urine in an attempt to define the difference between contamination and infection in midstream urine specimens. In a previous study, Marple (1941) had indicated the need to do quantitative colony counts on urine specimens, and Kass, in a series of publications, established the definition of bacteriuria as the presence of $>10^5$ bacteria per ml in two voided urine specimens (Norden & Kass 1968).

Most epidemiological studies of the significance of bacteriuria in pregnancy have used Kass's definition and, using his criteria, 4–15% of pregnant women in different studies have shown bacteriuria. It is noteworthy that 50% of patients with bacteriuria in pregnancy have upper urinary tract infection when localization studies are done (Fairley et al 1966). In individual patients, pregnancy bacteriuria localized to the bladder may ascend the ureter and show renal localization prior to the onset of acute pyelonephritis (Fig. 6.1.1–1) (Fairley 1971).

Kass noted that women with bacteriuria were very likely to develop pyelonephritis in pregnancy and that this could be prevented by treatment.

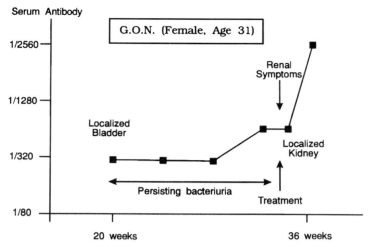

Fig. 6.1.1–1 Serum antibody titres against infecting organisms plotted against weeks of gestation in a woman with bladder bacteriuria identified by localization tests at 20 weeks which subsequently ascended the urethra and caused renal symptoms. Renal localization was confirmed on direct testing of ureteric specimens. A rise in antibody titre accompanied the renal infection. (From Fairley 1971, with permission.)

He also reported that the prematurity rate was increased in pregnancies complicated by bacteriuria (Kass 1959, 1960). In subsequent studies he reported that treatment of bacteriuria during pregnancy prevented prematurity (Kass 1965, Savage et al 1967, Elder et al 1967).

Numerous studies of bacteriuria in pregnancy followed Kass's original observations.

Without exception, studies confirmed that acute pyelonephritis is more frequent in women with bacteriuria and that this can be prevented by antibacterial treatment of the bacteriuria.

In our own study of 4000 pregnant women, 1.2% developed symptomatic infection, and 31% of bacteriuric women receiving placebo developed symptoms compared with 1.5% of bacteriuric women on antibacterial treatment (Table 6.1.1–1) (Kincaid-Smith 1964, Kincaid-Smith & Bullen 1965).

Following a series of similar studies in the early 1960s, screening for pregnancy bacteriuria became standard antenatal practice because of the unequivocal demonstration that antibacterial treatment of bacteriuria prevented acute pyelonephritis. A recent decision and cost analysis has confirmed the cost effectiveness of screening for asymptomatic bacteriuria in pregnancy (Wadland & Plante 1989).

The question of the association of prematurity

Table 6.1.1–1 Symptomatic urinary tract infection/pyelonephritis

	Total no.	Symptomatic infection	Percentage
No bacteriuria (at first antenatal visit)	4000	48	1.2
Placebo (bacteriuria at first antenatal visit)	60 (47)[†]	19 (19)	31 (40)
Treatment (bacteriuria at first antenatal visit)	64 (55)	1* (1)	1.5 (1.8)

† Patients with bacteria on two occasions
* Persistent bacteriuria

with bacteriuria has not been confirmed in all studies. Table 6.1.1–2 shows the results in a number of studies. In each study, except in the small study of Low, there were more premature infants recorded among bacteriuric than among non-bacteriuric pregnancies. In several studies, the prematurity rate in the bacteriuric population was more than double that in non-bacteriuric pregnancies. Perhaps the differences reflect some difference in the population studied.

Only Kass's group (Kass 1965, Savage et al 1967, Elder et al 1968) reported a reduction in prematurity using antibacterial treatment during pregnancy. In our study, in which 13.3% of bacteriuric women gave birth to premature infants

Table 6.1.1–2   Bacteriuria and prematurity (from Kincaid–Smith 1968 with permission)

Reference	Bacteriuric			Non-bacteriuric		
		Premature			Premature	
	Total	No.	%	Total	No.	%
Little*	265	33	8.7	4735	360	7.6
Kincaid-Smith & Bullen†	240	32	13.3	500	25	5.0
Whalley*	176	26	15	176	21	12
Norden & Kilpatrick*	114	17	15	109	14	7
Sleigh et al*	100	7	7	100	7	7
Kass*	95	26	27	1000	88	9
Stuart et al*	88	20	23	729	83	11
Low et al	80	5	6	690	49	8
Layton*	63	10	17	114	10	9
Totals	1221	166	13.6	9953	657	8.2

$\chi^2 = 10.827$ $P<0.001$

* Quoted by Whalley (1967).
† Quoted by Kincaid-Smith (1968)

compared with 5.0% of non-bacteriuric women, we were unable to reduce the rate of prematurity by treatment. We attributed prematurity to the high rate of underlying renal disease in our bacteriuric patients (Table 6.1.1–3). In our own study a high percentage of patients had underlying radiological abnormalities, most commonly reflux nephropathy, and in two studies in London (Williams et al 1965, Little 1966) there was a higher incidence of prematurity in women in whom infection was difficult to eradicate. Such patients commonly have underlying radiographic abnormalities (Kincaid-Smith & Bullen 1965, Williams et al 1965).

It is possible that this high rate of underlying renal disease in bacteriuric women was also a factor in the increased fetal loss (Table 6.1.1–4) and increased preeclampsia which we observed in bacteriuric women (Table 6.1.1–5).

Two other studies (Norden & Kilpatrick 1965, Stuart et al 1965) found a significantly higher incidence of preeclampsia in bacteriuric women but, as in our study, treatment of the bacteriuria did not reduce the incidence of preeclampsia.

Treatment also had no effect in reducing fetal loss in bacteriuric women in our study, perhaps because the fetal loss which often occurred in the second trimester was a reflection of the underlying renal disease indicated by radiographic lesions (Table 6.1.1–3).

Thus, in summary, bacteriuria in pregnancy is associated with a high risk of acute pyelonephritis

Table 6.1.1–3   Radiological findings — intravenous pyelogram in 134 of 200 patients

	No.	%
Normal	67	50
Chronic pyelonephritis (reflux nephropathy)	27	40.2
Calyceal abnormality, papillary necrosis or chronic pyelonephritis	11	8.2
Renal calculi	10	7.5
Duplex system (3 with localized chronic pyelonephritis)	3	4.5
Miscellaneous (e.g. marked hydronephrosis, tuberculosis, hypernephroma, >2 cm difference in kidney length)	16	11.9
Total	134	

Table 6.1.1–4 Fetal loss

	Total	Fetal loss at 13–27 weeks		Fetal loss at 28–40 weeks		Total fetal loss	
		No.	%	No.	%	No.	%
Non-bacteriuric	500	8	1.6	8	1.6	16	3.2
Bacteriuric	200	10	5	10	5	20	10
Treatment	64			4	6.2		
Placebo	60			4	6.6		
Treatment*	55			4	7.2		
Placebo*	47			4	8.5		
Treatment—free of bacteriuria until delivery	47			4	8.5		

*Excluding cases without bacteriuria on second count. Significant difference between non-bacteriuric and bacteriuric patients ($\chi^2 = 13.54$; $P<0.01$)

Table 6.1.1–5 Preeclamptic toxaemia

	Total	No.	%
Non-bacteriuric	500	30*	6
Bacteriuric	200	22*	11
Treatment	64	7	10.9
Placebo	60	7	11.6
Treatment[†]	55	6	10.9
Placebo[†]	47	6	12.7
Treatment — free of bacteriuria until delivery	47	6	12.7

[†]Excluding patients without bacteriuria on second count.
*Significant difference between non-bacteriuric and bacteriuric patients ($\chi^2 = 5.19$; $P<0.05$).

developing during pregnancy. There is unequivocal evidence from many studies that treatment of bacteriuria prevents the development of acute pyelonephritis. Some studies have shown an increase in prematurity, fetal loss and preeclampsia in women with bacteriuria; this may be due to the high prevalence of underlying renal disease such as reflux nephropathy and calculi which have been demonstrated in bacteriuric women in some studies.

6.1.2 Symptomatic acute cystitis

In our prospective study we found that no patient who had previously been documented to have asymptomatic bacteriuria developed symptomatic cystitis during pregnancy — each bacteriuric patient who subsequently developed symptoms had unequivocal clinical features of acute pyelonephritis (Kincaid-Smith & Bullen 1965).

Among women who had no bacteriuria on screening, 48 developed symptomatic infection which was acute cystitis in 16 and acute pyelonephritis in 32.

In non-pregnant women, acute cystitis is far more common than acute pyelonephritis and this apparent predisposition of pregnant women to develop renal rather than bladder symptoms is discussed under 6.1.3.

Although we have not done a formal study, and know of no other formal study, we have frequently observed individual patients who have troublesome recurrent acute cystitis when they are not pregnant but seem to have a remission from these symptoms during pregnancy. The predisposing factor in women who get recurrent symptoms of acute cystitis is colonization of the vulvovaginal area by urinary tract pathogens associated with bacterial adherence to vaginal cells (Stamey & Pfau 1970). Whether some factor or factors in pregnancy alter these predisposing factors is speculative. Stenquist et al (1989) showed an association between bacterial adhesion and renal infection in bacteriuria of pregnancy.

In one study in general practice (Gaymans et al 1976) symptomatic infections were more common during pregnancy than in non-pregnant women, but the authors did not state whether the symptomatic infections were cystitis or pyelonephritis.

6.1.3 Acute pyelonephritis

Acute pyelonephritis is one of the most frequent and most serious medical complications of pregnancy occurring in some 1–2% of pregnant women. In our prospective study we observed acute pyelonephritis in 0.8% of women without bacteriuria at the time of screening. Gilstrap et al (1981a) documented acute pyelonephritis in 2% of pregnant women.

Bacteriuria is present during pregnancy in some 4–7% of women (Stamey 1980) and 25–36% of these develop acute pyelonephritis; thus pregnant women have a considerably increased risk over non-pregnant women of developing acute pyelonephritis.

We observed that bacteriuria in pregnancy is usually accompanied by an increased urinary leucocyte count and that the count rises progressively to very high levels in the weeks before the onset of symptoms leading to an episode of acute pyelonephritis (Kincaid-Smith & Bullen 1965). The leucocyte count, like the bacterial count, usually falls after antibacterial treatment; if it does not fall, it is likely that there is an underlying lesion such as a calculus which will cause persisting infection (Kincaid-Smith & Bullen 1965).

The reason for the progressive rise in urinary leucocyte count in the weeks before acute pyelonephritis develops is not clear. 50% of pregnancy bacteriuria is localized to the bladder (Fairley et al 1966), and in those with a bladder localization the antibody titre against the infecting organism is low (Fairley 1971). When acute pyelonephritis develops in a patient with a previous bladder bacteriuria the site of infection changes from bladder to kidney and at the same time the serum antibody titre against the infecting organism rises (Fig. 6.1.1–1).

One of the abnormalities present during pregnancy is the so-called physiological dilatation of the ureter pelvis and calyces (Fig. 2.2–1). This change may play a part in the predisposition of the pregnant woman to acute pyelonephritis. In reports of acute pyelonephritis in pregnancy, before antibacterial drugs were available, rapid recovery often followed delivery (Falls 1923). Whereas pregnancy bacteriuria is localized to the bladder in 50% of all cases, when there is dilatation of the upper urinary tract the bacteriuria is always renal in localization and in unilateral dilatation is always on the side of the dilated ureter

(Fairley et al 1966). This observation strongly suggests that so-called 'physiological' dilatation of the urinary tract during pregnancy is one factor which predisposes to renal infection. A further interesting observation in relation to renal infection and pelvicalyceal dilatation is the recent finding of Twickler et al (1991) which showed significantly greater dilatation of the pelvis in women with acute pyelonephritis than in those with so-called physiological dilatation of pregnancy.

Acute pyelonephritis in pregnancy is a potentially life threatening illness which claimed many lives before antibiotics were available. Women with obstruction and infection are at particular risk and may develop septic shock which still causes deaths in women with acute pyelonephritis (Cunningham et al 1973).

Treatment of acute pyelonephritis of pregnancy must be prompt and, as the patient is often nauseated or vomiting, parenteral treatment is usually necessary.

Complete obstruction of the ureter at the pelvic brim may occur in women with acute pyelonephritis in pregnancy (Carey et al 1989). Calculi are one of the commonest lesions found in association with pregnancy bacteriuria and pyelonephritis (Kincaid-Smith & Bullen 1965, Bullen & Kincaid-Smith 1971) and may cause obstruction in pregnancy. Obstruction of the urinary tract may be relieved as part of the management of the acute pyelonephritis and is conveniently done by percutaneous nephrostomy through which a ureteric calculus can also be removed (Carey et al 1989).

Renal abscess or carbuncle may rarely occur as a complication of acute pyelonephritis of pregnancy (Moore & Gangai 1976, Soules et al 1976).

Recurrence of acute pyelonephritis during pregnancy is common and is likely to reflect an underlying lesion such as a calculus. This occurred in 10% of 99 cases studied by Cunningham et al (1973).

Maternal urinary tract infections predispose to prematurity and neonatal deaths (Naeye 1979); however, this excess mortality is accounted for by urinary tract infections within 15 days of delivery.

In some series, no adverse fetal or neonatal effects of acute pyelonephritis have been recorded (Cunningham et al 1973, Gilstrap et al 1981b, Yuan-Da Fan et al 1987).

REFERENCES

Albeck V 1907 Bakteriurie und Pyurie bei Schwangeren und Gebärenden. Zeitschrift fur Geburtshilfe und Gynaekologie 60: 466–537

Bullen M, Kincaid-Smith P 1971 Asymptomatic pregnancy bacteriuria — a follow-up study 4–7 years after delivery. In: P Kincaid-Smith, K F Fairley (eds) Renal infection and renal scarring. Mercedes Publishing, Melbourne, pp 33–39

Carey M P, Ihle B U, Woodwood C S et al 1989 Ureteric obstruction by the gravid uterus. Australian and New Zealand Journal of Obstetrics and Gynaecology 29: 308–313

Cunningham F G, Morris G B, Mickal A 1973 Acute pyelonephritis of pregnancy: a clinical review. Obstetrics and Gynecology 42: 112–116

Dodds G 1931 Bacteriuria in pregnancy. Labour and the puerperium. Journal of Obstetrics and Gynaecology of the British Empire 38: 773–787

Elder H A, Santamarina B A G, Smith S et al 1967 Excess prematurity in tetracycline-treated bacteriuric patients whose infection persisted or returned. Antimicrobial agents. Chemotherapy 7: 101–109

Fairley K F 1971 The routine determination of the site of infection in the investigation of patients with urinary tract infection. In: P Kincaid-Smith, K F Fairley (eds) Renal infection and renal scarring. Mercedes Publishing, Melbourne, pp 107–116

Fairley K F, Bond A G, Adey FD et al 1966 The site of infection in pregnancy bacteriuria. Lancet 1: 939–941

Falls F H 1923 A contribution to the study of pyelitis in pregnancy. Journal of the American Medical Association 81: 1590–1593

Gaymans R, Valkenburg H A, Haverkorn M J et al 1976 A prospective study of urinary-tract infections in a Dutch general practice. Lancet 2: 674

Gilstrap L C, Cunningham F G, Whalley P J 1981a Acute pyelonephritis in pregnancy: an interoceptive study of 565 women. Obstetrics and Gynecology 65: 409–413

Gilstrap L C, Leveno K J, Cunningham F G et al 1981b Renal infection and pregnancy outcome. American Journal of Obstetrics and Gynecology 141: 709–716

Kass E H 1955 Chemotherapeutic and antibiotic drugs in the management of infections of the urinary tract. American Journal of Medicine 18: 764–781

Kass E H 1959 Bacteriuria and pyelonephritis of pregnancy. Transactions of the Association of American Physicians 72: 257–264

Kass E H 1960 Bacteriuria and pyelonephritis of pregnancy. Archives of Internal Medicine 105: 194–198

Kass E H 1965 The significance of bacteriuria in preventive medicine. In: E H Kass (ed) Progress in pyelonephritis. F A Davis, Baltimore, pp 3–10

Kincaid-Smith P 1964 Bacteriuria in pregnancy. In: E H Kass (ed) Progress in glomerulonephritis. F A. Davis, Baltimore pp 11–26

Kincaid-Smith P, Bullen M 1965 Bacteriuria in pregnancy. Lancet 1: 395–399

Kincaid-Smith P 1968 Bacteriuria and urinary infection in pregnancy. Clinical Obstetrics and Gynecology 11: 533–549

Little P J 1966 The incidence of urinary infection in 5,000 pregnant women. Lancet 2: 925–928

Low J A, Johnson E E, McBride R L et al 1964 The significance of asymptomatic bacteriuria in the normal obstetric patient. American Journal of Obstetric Gynecology 90: 897–906

Marple C 1941 The frequency and character of urinary tract infections in an unselected group of women. Annals of Internal Medicine 14: 2220–2239

Moore C A, Gangai M P 1967 Renal cortical abscess. Journal of Urology 98: 303–306

Naeye R L 1979 Causes of the excessive rates of perinatal mortality and prematurity in pregnancies complicated by maternal urinary-tract infections. New England Journal of Medicine 300: 819–823

Norden C W, Kass E H 1968 Bacteriuria of pregnancy — a critical appraisal. Annual Review of Medicine 19: 431–470

Norden C W, Kilpatrick W 1965 Bacteriuria in pregnancy. In: E H Kass (ed) Progress in glomerulonephritis. F A Davis, Baltimore, pp 64–72

Rayer P 1839–1841 Traite des maladies des reins et des alterations de la secretion urinaire. J B Baillière, Paris, vol II: pp 399–407

Reblaub T 1892 Cong Franc Chir (Paris) 6: 110–120

Savage W, Haji S N, Kass EH 1967 Demographic and prognostic characteristics of bacteriuria in pregnancy. Medicine 46: 385–407

Sleigh J D, Robertson J G, Isdale M H 1964 Asymptomatic bacteriuria in pregnancy. Journal of Obstetrics and Gynaecology of the British Commonwealth 71: 74–81

Soules M R, Stables D P, Pfister R R 1976 Renal carbuncle; unusual cause of post-partum febrile morbidity. Journal of Reproductive Medicine 16: 97–101

Stamey T A (ed) 1980 Pathogenesis and treatment of urinary tract infections. Williams & Wilkins, Baltimore, p 210–289

Stamey T A, Pfau A 1970 Urinary infections: a selective review and some observations. California Medicine 113: 16–35

Stenqvist K, Lidin-Janson G, Sandberg T et al 1989 Bacterial adhesion as an indicator of renal involvement in bacteriuria of pregnancy. Scandinavian Journal of Infectious Diseases 21: 193–199

Stuart K L, Cummins G T M, Chin W 1965 Bacteriuria, prematurity, and the hypertensive disorders of pregnancy. British Medical Journal 1: 554–556

Twickler D, Little B B, Satin A J et al 1991 Renal pelvicalyceal dilation in antepartum pyelonephritis: ultrasonographic findings. American Journal of Obstetrics and Gynecology 165: 1115–11159

Wadland W C, Plante D A 1989 Screening for asymptomatic bacteriuria in pregnancy: a decision and cost analysis. Journal of Family Practice 29: 372–376

Whalley P 1967 Bacteriuria of pregnancy. American Journal of Obstetrics and Gynecology 97: 723–738

Williams J D, Brumfitt W, Leight D et al 1965 Eradication of bacteriuria in pregnancy by a short course of chemotherapy. Lancet 1: 831

Yuan-Da Fan, Pastorek J G, Miller J M et al 1987 Acute pyelonephritis in pregnancy. American Journal of Perinatology 4: 324–326

6.2 RENAL CALCULI

Renal calculi are relatively uncommon in women

of child bearing age. They may, however, cause serious complications in pregnancy when associated with infection and particularly when both infection and obstruction are present.

Calculi were detected in 7.5% of women who were found to have bacteriuria in pregnancy on screening (Kincaid-Smith & Bullen 1964, 1965). In the same series a further 3% of women developed renal calculi during the 6 months following delivery (Bullen & Kincaid-Smith 1971).

The only reduction in renal size observed over 4–6 years' follow up of women with bacteriuria of pregnancy was a 3cm reduction in renal length in 1 patient following obstruction by a ureteric calculus (Bullen & Kincaid-Smith 1971). The size reduction continued to progress for 3 years following pregnancy, in spite of removal of the calculus soon after its detection in the early postpartum period. In contrast, no further reduction in size or increase in scarring was noted in women with reflux nephropathy in this series.

Not only are urinary tract calculi found in association with bacteriuria in pregnancy but there is also an increase in urinary infection in pregnant women with calculi (Coe et al 1978).

The incidence of stone disease during pregnancy is difficult to assess because of the selective nature of most reports on this topic. In our study, urinary tract calculi were found in 10 women with bacteriuria derived from a screened population of 4000, i.e. 0.25% of women had calculi. No radiological studies were performed in women who did not have bacteriuria, so that our study could have underestimated the incidence of calculi. Careful midstream urine examinations were done, however, and we would have investigated any patient with microscopic haematuria or pyuria — the urine findings which usually accompany calculi. This figure of 0.25% is in the middle range of that in other studies, which vary from 0.03% to 0.53% (Coe et al 1978, Miller & Kakkis 1982, Horowitz & Schmidt 1985).

In addition to infection, another factor in pregnancy which could lead to an increase in stone formation is the dilatation of the ureter, pelvis and calyces which is accompanied by a decrease in ureteric peristalsis (Waltzer 1981). Although Coe et al (1978) found no evidence of an increased incidence of calculi in pregnancy, studies which we have carried out in individual patients would suggest that existing calculi may increase considerably in size during the course of one pregnancy. We have observed this in individual patients with struvite calculi, uric acid calculi and cystine calculi, where rapid stone growth has resulted in staghorn calculi developing during pregnancy. Struvite stone growth occurs in association with infection but other factors, perhaps the stasis within the urinary tract, must be responsible for the increase in size of uric acid and cystine calculi during pregnancy.

Renal colic is the commonest non-obstetric cause of abdominal pain requiring hospitalization during pregnancy (Folger 1955).

Ultrasound is now the preferred technique used to assess the presence of ureteric obstruction and the site of obstruction. This technique does not always achieve adequate visualization of the calculus because the majority are in the lower ureter (Horowitz & Schmidt 1985).

Table 6.2–1 derived from the review by Maikranz et al (1987) summarizes the findings in recent reports of renal calculi in pregnancy. Three quarters of the renal calculi were passed spontaneously, only a small number requiring intervention.

The indications for intervention during pregnancy include continuing renal colic, a high grade of obstruction or obstruction with infection.

Percutaneous nephrostomy to relieve the obstruction may be all that is required; alternatively internal ureteric stents can be used (Loughlin & Bailey 1986). Internal stents may become encrusted and lead to both pyelonephritis (Abber & Kahn 1983) and further stone formation (Spirnak & Resnick 1985, Goldfarb et al 1989). Encrustation may develop over as short a period as 2–3 weeks.

Percutaneous removal of ureteric calculi can be performed through a nephrostomy with safety in pregnancy (Fig. 6.2–1); however, some advise that this should be delayed until the postpartum period (Rodriguez & Klein 1988).

The availability of ureteroscopic and percutaneous nephrostomy techniques mean that open surgical procedures are now rarely if ever necessary during pregnancy.

Calculi which present during pregnancy should

Table 6.2–1   The passage of kidney stones (modified from Maikranz et al, 1987)

Source	n[*]	Stones passed spontaneously	Non-operative[†] procedures	Operative procedures	Other[†]
Coe et al 1978	20 (15)	20	0	0	0
Drago et al 1982	12 (9)	9	1	2	0
Horowitz & Schmidt 1985	17 (17)	5	10	2	0
Jones et al 1978	21 (20)	12	2 (1¶)	5 (4¶)	2
Lattanzie & Cook 1980	11 (11)	7	2	0	2
Perreault et al 1982	19 (19)	14	0	4 (1¶)	0

[*]No. of stones reported, no. of pregnancies in parentheses.
[†]Cystoscopy, percutaneous nephrostomy or basket extraction.
[†] Patients either lost to follow-up or without clinical evidence of stone passage.
¶ No. of procedures done post partum.

be followed up in the same way as in those in non-pregnant women in terms of stone analysis and investigation for underlying predisposing causes. We find that we can identify a cause in most patients and having done so can usually prevent recurrence.

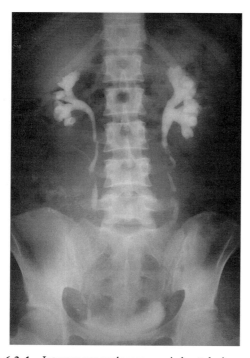

Fig. 6.2–1   Intravenous pyelogram carried out during pregnancy in a woman presenting with severe recurrent left pyelonephritis. The ureteric calculus demonstrated in the left ureter is causing incomplete obstruction and was removed by basket extraction through a percutaneous nephrostomy.

The most frequent calculi which we have encountered during pregnancy are infection or struvite stones in which the calculus and its fragments contain the causative urea splitting organism, most frequently *Proteus mirabilis*. The infection cannot be eradicated and patients require full dose suppressive antibiotic treatment during pregnancy to prevent persistent infection and recurrent episodes of acute pyelonephritis. After the pregnancy, complete removal of the calculus and its fragments should be undertaken and the urine must be maintained sterile with the patient off any antibiotics before a subsequent pregnancy is undertaken. If the urine remains infected the likely cause is persistence of small stone fragments and these can be dissolved by a substance called renacidin which can be given through a nephrostomy catheter (Dretler et al 1979).

Calcium oxalate stones are often associated with idiopathic hypercalciuria and urine calcium excretion increases during pregnancy (Pederson et al 1984). In non-pregnant women thiazides are commonly used to prevent stone recurrence; however, some recommend that thiazide administration should cease during pregnancy. As discussed in 5.4 there is really no evidence that thiazides are harmful in pregnancy.

Recurrent uric acid calculi are often treated with allopurinol; however, this drug has complex metabolic effects and should probably be ceased during pregnancy. Simple increased urine output and alkalization of the urine will usually prevent uric acid calculus formation during pregnancy.

Cystine stones may be troublesome to manage during pregnancy (Gregory & Mansell 1983). We have observed a considerable increase in cystine stone size during pregnancy. Penicillamine has teratogenic effects in animals and an increase in a disease of elastic tissue has been reported in humans. It is best avoided during pregnancy when very high urine volumes may be required to lower urine cystine concentrations and prevent an increase in the number and size of calculi.

REFERENCES

Abber J C, Kahn R J 1983 Pyelonephritis from severe encrustation on silicone ureteral stents: management. Journal of Urology 130: 763–764

Bullen M, Kincaid-Smith P 1971 Asymptomatic pregnancy bacteriuria — a follow-up study 4–7 years after delivery. In: P Kincaid-Smith, K F Fairley (eds) Renal infection and renal scarring. Mercedes Publishing, Melbourne, pp 33–39

Coe F L, Parks J H, Lindheimer M D 1978 Nephrolithiasis during pregnancy. New England Journal of Medicine 298: 324–326

Drago J R, Rohner T J, Chez R A 1982 Management of urinary calculi in pregnancy. Urology 20: 578–581

Dretler S P, Pfister R C, Newhouse J H 1979 Renal-stone dissolution via percutaneous nephrostomy. New England Journal of Medicine 300: 341–343

Folger G K 1955 Pain and pregnancy: treatment of painful states complicating pregnancy, with particular emphasis on urinary calculi. Obstetrics and Gynecology 5: 513–518

Goldfarb R A, Neerhut G J, Lederer E 1989 Management of acute hydronephrosis of pregnancy by ureteral stenting: risk of stone formation. Journal of Urology 141: 921–922

Gregory M C, Mansell M A 1983 Pregnancy and cystinuria. Lancet 2: 1158–1160

Horowitz E, Schmidt J D 1985 Renal calculi in pregnancy. Clinical Obstetrics and Gynecology 28: 324–338

Jones W A, Correa Jr R J, Ansell J S 1978 Urolithiasis associated with pregnancy. Journal of Urology 122: 333–338

Kincaid-Smith P, Bullen M 1964 Bacteriuria in pregnancy. In: E H Kass (ed) Progress in pyelonephritis. F A Davis, Philadelphia, pp 11–26

Kincaid-Smith P, Bullen M 1965 Bacteriuria in pregnancy. Lancet 1: 395–399

Lattanzi D R, Cook W A 1980 Urinary calculi in pregnancy. Obstetrics and Gynecology 56:462–466

Loughlin K R, Bailey RB 1986 Internal ureteral stents for conservative management of ureteral calculi during pregnancy. New England Journal of Medicine 315: 1647–1649

Maikranz P, Coe F L, Parks J H et al MD 1987 Nephrolithiasis and gestation. Baillières Clinical Obstetrics and Gynaecology 1: 909–919

Miller R D, Kakkis J 1982 Prognosis, management and outcome of obstructive renal disease in pregnancy. Journal of Reproductive Medicine 28: 199–201

Pederson E B, Johannesen P, Kristensen S et al 1984 Calcium, parathyroid hormone and calcitonin in normal pregnancy and preeclampsia. Gynecologic and Obstetric Investigation 18: 156–164

Perreault J P, Paquin JM, Faucher R et al 1982 Urinary calculi in pregnancy. Canadian Journal of Surgery 25: 453–454

Rodriguez P N, Klein A S 1988 Management of urolithiasis during pregnancy. Surgery, Gynecology and Obstetrics 166: 103–106

Spirnak J P, Resnick M I 1985 Stone formation as a complication of indwelling ureteral stents: a report of 5 cases. Journal of Urology 134: 349–351

Waltzer W C 1981 The urinary tract in pregnancy. Journal of Urology 125: 271–276

6.3 ACUTE RENAL FAILURE

The frequency of acute renal failure during pregnancy and in the early postpartum period suggests that the kidney is particularly susceptible to this complication during pregnancy. The four types of acute renal failure associated with pregnancy, namely prerenal failure, acute tubular necrosis, cortical necrosis and thrombotic microangiopathy, are different in terms of pathology and prognosis and the underlying pathophysiological mechanisms also differ; in each case, however, pregnancy seems to be a factor which predisposes to the development of acute renal failure. A number of conditions are associated with acute renal failure in pregnancy. These are listed in Table 6.3–1.

6.3.1. Prerenal failure and acute tubular necrosis

Prerenal acute renal failure in which oliguria is related to prerenal factors such as decreased intravascular volume is seen as a complication of preeclampsia. Restoration of a normal urine output in such patients has been achieved using low dose dopamine (2 mg/kg/min), demonstrating

Table 6.3–1   Conditions associated with acute renal failure in pregnancy

Clinical condition	Usual pathology
Septic abortion	Acute tubuar necrosis
Abruptio placentae	Cortical necrosis
Severe preeclampsia	Prerenal failure or acute tubular necrosis
Acute fatty liver	Prerenal failure or acute tubular necrosis
Acute pyelonephritis	Acute tubular necrosis
Prolonged fetal death in utero	Cortical necrosis
Malignant hypertension	Thrombotic microangiopathy
Lupus anticoagulant	Thrombotic microangiopathy

that it is due to haemodynamic factors and not established acute tubular necrosis.

The major obstetric cause of acute tubular necrosis during pregnancy in the early series treated by dialysis was septic abortion (Kennedy et al 1973, Knapp & Hellman 1959, Kincaid-Smith & Fairley 1981). *Clostridium welchii* infections were prominent among the causes of sepsis and until dialysis became available the mortality in these cases was extremely high.

Legalization of abortion and its availability as a procedure performed under aseptic conditions in hospital has almost eliminated septic abortion as a cause of acute tubular necrosis in most of the developed world. In Melbourne over a 20-year period pregnancy associated acute renal failure was reduced by a factor of four to five (Kincaid-Smith & Fairley 1981), and in Dublin a six-fold reduction was recorded (Donohue 1983).

Acute tubular necrosis usually recovers completely. The period of renal failure, which is usually associated with oliguria but occasionally polyuria, usually lasts 2 weeks but occasionally may last as long as 4 weeks. In cases with more prolonged periods of oliguric renal failure, considerable loss of fluid and electrolytes may occur during the diuretic phase. Full recovery of renal function is usual with no residual abnormalities. Maternal mortality in published series remains high, estimated as 16.8% by Finn (1983).

6.3.2 Acute cortical necrosis

The majority of recorded cases of acute cortical necrosis have occurred during pregnancy. Classically acute cortical necrosis occurs as a complication of abruptio placentae with concealed accidental haemorrhage.

The association of pregnancy and acute cortical necrosis was recognized during the last century. The first British description is often attributed to Bradford & Lawrence (1898). Reading this description of a case which occurred in the early postpartum period, there are features such as the severe anaemia and the extensive thrombosis in interlobular arteries which suggest that this may have been a case of thrombotic microangiopathy. Patchy cortical necrosis can occur in postpartum renal failure associated with

thrombotic microangiopathy (Counihan & Doniach 1954) and sometimes there is confusion between this diagnosis and that of classical cortical necrosis associated with concealed accidental haemorrhage (Sheehan & Moore 1952).

Cortical necrosis may be accompanied by a defibrination syndrome and disseminated intravascular coagulation. These coagulation disorders themselves constitute a life threatening disorder.

The renal lesion of acute cortical necrosis may affect 90% or more of the renal cortex or it may be patchy leaving large areas of surviving cortical tissue. The latter cases usually recover adequate renal function, although scarring of the renal cortex due to fibrosis in necrotic areas persists (Kincaid-Smith 1975). A wide range of different degrees of partial recovery of renal function is possible following acute cortical necrosis. The survival of surprisingly small areas of renal cortex can permit recovery independent of dialysis (Kincaid-Smith et al 1967). In patients who are initially placed on maintenance dialysis in the belief that recovery will not occur, it may be possible to cease dialysis weeks or months later.

6.3.3 Acute thrombotic microangiopathy

The lesions which occur in association with a microangiopathic haemolytic anaemia, thrombocytopenia and other features of disseminated intervascular coagulation do not differ greatly from those seen in acute cortical necrosis. As noted above, it is difficult to be sure if Bradford & Lawrence (1898) described the first case of postpartum renal failure due to thrombotic microangiopathy or whether this was the first description of cortical necrosis — probably it was the latter. Early reports by McKelvey & MacMahon (1935) and Zimmerman & Peters (1937) described the vascular lesions of malignant hypertension in women who died of preeclampsia. Zimmerman & Peters (1937) made a point of emphasizing the severity of vascular lesions which contrasted with 'benign' hypertension noted clinically. These two reports were probably examples of pregnancy associated thrombotic microangiopathy.

Counihan & Doniach (1954) described 2 cases which are in every respect typical of the syndrome which is characterized by a renal failure associated with microangiopathic haemolytic anaemia, subsequent development of severe hypertension and renal lesions resembling those seen in the haemolytic uraemic syndrome.

Reisfield (1959) described 2 cases of thrombotic microangiopathy occurring in pregnancy in which the renal lesions consisted of hyaline thrombi in glomeruli but where renal function was only mildly impaired. A similar case was recorded by Solomon et al (1963). Scheer & Jones (1967) described further cases resembling those reported by Counihan & Doniach (1954); and Robson et al (1968), who titled this 'a new syndrome', also described essentially similar cases of postpartum renal failure and thrombotic microangiopathy.

Many subsequent reports have appeared. It should be noted that identical lesions and a similar clinical course may occur in patients taking oral contraceptive agents (Schoolwerth et al 1976).

We have described this syndrome in association with a circulating lupus anticoagulant (Kincaid-Smith et al 1988).

The mortality rate of thrombotic microangiopathy occurring in pregnancy or in the early postpartum period has been very high. The haematological abnormalities associated with this syndrome are thrombocytopenia, raised fibrin degradation products and a microangiopathic haemolytic anaemia.

Some degree of recovery of renal function was achieved using heparin and antiplatelet agents (Kincaid-Smith 1973, Donadio & Holley 1974), but more recently plasma exchange has proved very effective (Rock et al 1991, Bell et al 1991).

It had been suggested that the underlying mechanism predisposing to thrombotic microangiopathy was the lack of some antithrombotic component of plasma such as prostacyclin, and plasma infusion had a vogue as a therapeutic method (Moake et al 1985). A recent publication clearly establishes that plasma exchange is more effective than plasma infusion in the treatment of thrombotic microangiopathies and thrombotic thrombocytopenia (Rock et al 1991). Not only

was short term recovery more frequent in patients treated by plasma exchange (47% in plasma exchange groups and 25% in plasma infusion groups) but the long term survival at 6 months was significantly better.

Endothelial cell damage is assumed to be the primary abnormality in the thrombotic microangiopathies, unusually large von Willebrand factor multimers form in association with the endothelial damage and they may be associated with platelet thrombi in the renal circulation (Moake & MacPherson 1989).

These unusually large von Willebrand factor multimers can be removed by plasma exchange, and this may be one mechanism whereby plasma exchange conveys benefit. Most patients require frequent exchanges daily or on alternate days in the initial 2 weeks (Bell et al 1991).

The renal lesion seen in this form of acute renal failure consists of thrombi in afferent arterioles (Fig. 6.3.3–1) and glomerular capillaries (Fig. 6.3.3–2). Interlobular arteries may also show thrombi. These platelet and fibrin thrombi

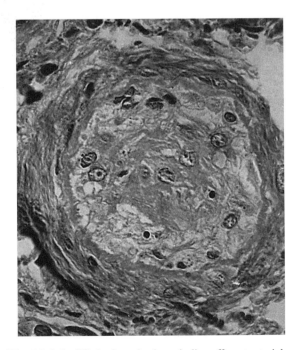

Fig. 6.3.3–1 Fibrin thrombosis occluding afferent arteriole in a case of postpartum renal failure due to thrombotic microangiopathy.

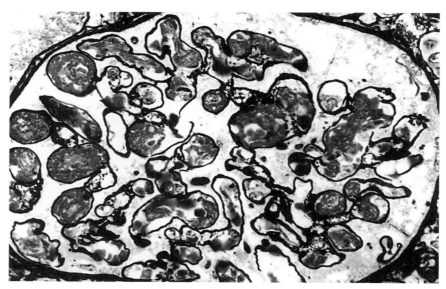

Fig. 6.3.3–2   Fibrin thrombi occluding many glomerular capillaries in a biopsy from a patient with renal failure due to acute thrombotic microangiopathy during pregnancy.

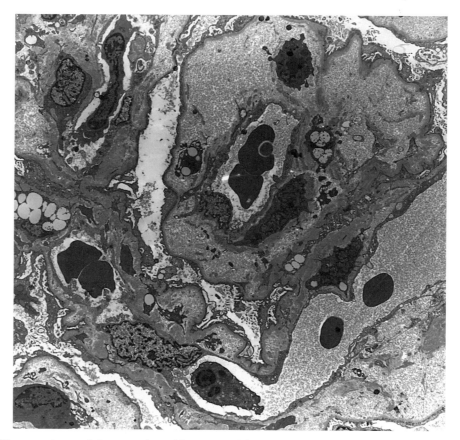

Fig. 6.3.3–3   Electron micrograph from a patient with acute renal failure due to thrombotic microangiopathy during pregnancy. Characteristic large translucent subendothelial deposits are present in glomerular capillaries.

are rapidly replaced by cellular intimal proliferation in interlobular arteries and arterioles. Very characteristic lesions are seen on electron microscopy in the glomeruli. Typical translucent sub- endothelial deposits (Fig. 6.3.3–3) are seen in the acute stage. Reduplication of basement membrane or double contours develop early (Fig. 6.3.3–4) but may persist for months or years after the

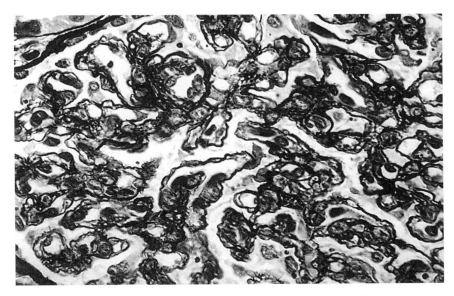

Fig. 6.3.3–4   Diffuse double contours in glomerular capillaries in a biopsy from a patient with postpartum renal failure and thrombotic microangiopathy.

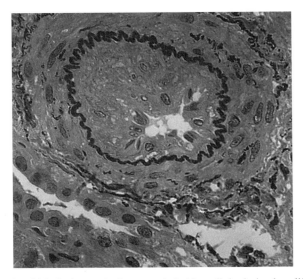

Fig. 6.3.3–5   Interlobular artery in which the lumen is almost occluded by cellular intimal proliferation in a biopsy taken weeks after an episode of acute renal failure due to thrombotic microangiopathy in pregnancy.

acute episode. Late arterial lesions consist of narrowing of interlobular arteries by fibroelastic or cellular intimal hyperplasia (Fig. 6.3.3–5). These may persist for as long as 10 years after the acute episode (Kincaid-Smith et al 1988).

Most women recovering from this form of acute renal failure have permanent persisting impairment of renal function. A recent study of children with the haemolytic uraemic syndrome, in which the pathological lesions are very similar to those seen in pregnancy associated thrombotic microangiopathy, shows persisting abnormalities in many children; 31% of children had protein-uria, 18% impaired renal function and 10% had hypertension at a mean time of 8.5 years after the acute episode (Fitzpatrick et al 1991). It is likely that women who recover following treatment of pregnancy associated thrombotic microangiopathy have more serious long term renal abnormalities than those in children where the haemolytic uraemic syndrome often recovers spontaneously and where the long term renal function has previously been reported as normal (Perelstein et al 1991).

REFERENCES

Bell W R, Braine H G, Ness P M et al 1991 Improved survival in thrombotic thrombocytopenic purpura–haemolytic uraemic syndrome: clinical experience in 108 patients. New England Journal of Medicine 325: 398–403

Bradford J R, Lawrence T W P 1898 Endarteritis of the renal arteries, causing necrosis of the entire cortex of both kidneys. Journal of Pathology and Bacteriology 5: 195–201

Counihan T B, Doniach I 1954 Malignant hypertension supervening rapidly on pre–eclampsia. Journal of Obstetrics and Gynaecology of the British Empire 56: 449–453

Donadio J V, Holley K E 1974 Postpartum acute renal failure: recovery after heparin therapy. American Journal of Obstetrics and Gynecology 118: 510–516

Donohoe J F 1983 Acute bilateral cortical necrosis. In: B M Brenner, J M Lazarus (eds) Acute renal failure. W B Saunders, Philadelphia, pp 252–268

Finn W F 1983 Recovery from acute renal failure. In: B M Brenner, J M Lazarus (eds) Acute renal failure. W B Saunders, Philadelphia, pp 252–268

Fitzpatrick M M, Shah V, Trompeter R S et al 1991 Long term renal outcome of childhood haemolytic uraemic syndrome. British Medical Journal 303: 489–492

Kennedy A C, Burton J A, Luke R G et al 1973 Factors affecting the prognosis in acute renal failure. Quarterly Journal of Medicine 42: 73–86

Kincaid-Smith P 1973 The similarity of lesions and underlying mechanism in pre-eclamptic toxaemia and postpartum renal failure. Studies in the acute stage and during follow-up. In: P Kincaid-Smith, T H Mathew, E L Becker (eds) Glomerulonephritis. Wiley, New York, pp 1047–1056

Kincaid-Smith P (ed) 1975 The kidney — a clinicopatho-logical study. Blackwell Scientific, Oxford, p 353

Kincaid-Smith P, Fairley K F 1981 The changing spectrum of acute renal failure in pregnancy and the post-partum period. Contributions to Nephrology 25: 159–165

Kincaid-Smith P, Fairley K F, Bullen M 1967 Kidney disease and pregnancy. Medical Journal of Australia 2: 1155–1159

Kincaid-Smith P, Fairley K F, Kloss M 1988 Lupus anticoagulant associated with renal thrombotic microangiopathy and pregnancy related renal failure. Quarterly Journal of Medicine (New Series 69) 258: 795–815

Knapp R C, Hellman L H 1959 Acute renal failure in pregnancy. American Journal of Obstetrics and Gynecology 78: 570–577

McKelvey J L, MacMahon H E 1935 A study of the lesions in the vascular system in fatal cases of chronic nephritic toxaemia of pregnancy. Surgery, Gynecology and Obstetrics 60: 1–18

Moake J L, McPherson P D 1989 Abnormalities of von Willebrand factor multimers in thrombotic thrombocytopenic purpura and the hemolytic–uremic syndrome. American Journal of Medicine 87 (suppl): 9–15

Moake J L, Byrnes J J, Troll J H et al 1985 Effects of fresh-frozen plasma and its cryosupernatant fraction on von Willebrand factor multimeric forms in chronic relapsing thrombotic thrombocytopenic purpura. Blood 65: 1232–1236

Perelstein E M, Grunfeld B G, Simsolo R B et al 1991 Renal functional reserve compared in haemolytic uraemic syndrome and single kidney. Archives of Disease in Childhood 65: 728–731

Reisfield D R 1959 Thrombotic thrombocytopenic purpura and pregnancy. Obstetrical and Gynecological Survey 14: 303–321

Rock G A, Shumak K H, Buskard N A et al and the Canadian Apheresis Study Group 1991 Comparison of plasma exchange with plasma infusion in the treatment of thrombotic thrombocytopenic purpura. New England Journal of Medicine 325: 393–397

Robson J S, Martin A M, Ruckley V A et al 1968 Irreversible postpartum renal failure: a new syndrome. Quarterly Journal of Medicine 37: 423–435

Schoolwerth A C, Sandler R S, Klahr S et al 1976 Nephrosclerosis postpartum and in women taking oral contraceptives. Archives of Internal Medicine 136: 178–185

Sheehan H L, Moore H C 1952 Renal cortical necrosis and the kidney of concealed accidental haemorrhage. Blackwell, Oxford

Scheer R L, Jones D B 1967 Malignant nephrosclerosis in women postpartum: a note on microangiopathic hemolytic anaemia. Journal of the American Medical Association 201: 106–110

Solomon W, Turner D S, Block C et al 1963 Thrombotic thrombocytopenic purpura in pregnancy. Journal of the American Medical Association 184: 587–590

Zimmerman H M, Peters J P 1937 Pathology of pregnancy toxaemias. Journal of Clinical Investigation 16: 397–420

6.4 PREGNANCY IN WOMEN WITH ECTOPIC KIDNEYS, IN WOMEN WHO HAVE UNDERGONE MAJOR URINARY TRACT DIVERSION AND IN WOMEN WITH OBSTRUCTION OF THE URINARY TRACT

6.4.1 Ectopic kidney

The influence of ectopic kidneys on the course of pregnancy depends upon the site of the ectopic kidney. These may be high (above the second lumbar vertebra), low (between the iliac crest and third lumbar vertebra), iliolumbar (over the iliac crest), iliac (in the iliac fossa) and pelvic (within the pelvis) (Eisendrath & Rolnick 1938).

It is the pelvic ectopic kidney which may be of concern to the obstetrician, and a single pelvic kidney, although rare, is of particular concern (Lowsley & Menning 1944). Pelvic kidneys may obstruct labour and require caesarean section, and in the past even more dramatic surgery such as nephrectomy has sometimes been carried out during pregnancy (Anderson et al 1949). The results in pregnancy prior to 1948 were associated with a high rate of fetal loss and a maternal mortality of 10% (Anderson et al 1949).

In some cases the pelvic ectopic kidney moves from the pelvis to a site above the pelvic rim during pregnancy (Fig. 6.4.1–1). In such cases pregnancy may proceed uneventfully. No recent review of results in women with ectopic kidneys has been found, but with prior knowledge of the anomaly caesarian section is usually carried out and the maternal and fetal outcome is much better than that recorded by Anderson et al (1949).

6.4.2 Pregnancy after major surgical diversion of the urinary tract

Ureterosigmoid anastomosis as a method of urinary tract diversion has been largely replaced by anastomosis of ureters into an ileal loop and more recently by the Kock pouch, a continent ileum reservoir (Kock et al 1978).

A review of reports in the literature of pregnancy in women who have undergone such procedures (Vordermark 1990) shows that complications of pregnancy are largely confined to

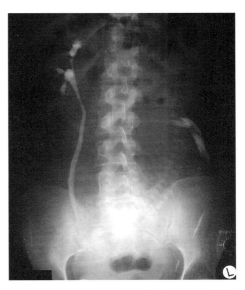

Fig. 6.4.1–1 Radiograph showing displacement of left pelvic kidney to a position above the pelvic brim by the fetal head.

local complications within the urinary tract and to infections. In Vordermark's report (1990) 15 of the 18 pregnancies resulted in full term, healthy infants; 8 of 15 were delivered by caesarian section. 4 pregnancies were complicated by recurrent urinary tract infection; 1 of these, in which *Proteus mirabilis* was the infecting organism, showed a progressive decline in renal function to a serum creatinine level of 1.9 mg/100 ml. Premature delivery in this patient resulted in a 1220 g infant which died. Two women developed urinary retention during pregnancy.

Hyperchloraemic acidosis, which is a feature of ureterosigmoid anastomosis, may worsen during pregnancy (Killan et al 1967).

One patient with an ileal loop urinary diversion developed complete obstruction of the ureters during pregnancy requiring a percutaneous nephrostomy (Laverson et al 1984).

6.4.3 Obstruction of the urinary tract

Although bilateral obstruction of the urinary tract with oliguria and deteriorating renal function rarely occurs as a complication of pregnancy (Lewis et al 1985), it is difficult to assess how commonly unilateral ureteric obstruction occurs.

Obstruction by ureteric calculi and obstruction by the gravid uterus at the pelvic brim are the two common causes of ureteric obstruction during pregnancy. The management of renal calculi is discussed in 6.2.

The diagnosis of ureteric obstruction by the pelvic brim is easy when it is bilateral because of the accompanying anuria and deterioration of renal funtion, but diagnosis of unilateral obstruction in one kidney is seldom made and may be much more frequent than bilateral obstruction. The diagnosis of unilateral obstruction is more commonly made in patients presenting with symptoms of loin pain and fever, and percutaneous nephrostomy has been used to reduce obstruction in such cases (Hinwood & Mahire 1991).

In a study of 76 patients in which ultrasound was combined with renography, a maximal anteroposterior diameter of the renal pelvis of 17 mm or above was found to be associated with complete ureteric obstruction in 43% of all cases. All those with an anteroposterior diameter above 29 mm were completely obstructed (Muller-Suur & Tyden 1985). This provides a useful guide to the likelihood of complete obstruction and is particularly useful in unilateral obstruction.

Twickler et al (1991) have shown that the degree of pelvicalyceal dilatation is greater in patients with pyelonephritis than in so-called physiological dilatation. The mean measurement of an anteroposterior diameter of 17 mm in patients with pyelonephritis in Twickler's study suggests that many of Muller-Suur & Tyden's patients may have been completely obstructed.

It is likely that the ready availability of ultrasound and its frequent use in pregnancy will lead to increasing recognition of obstruction of the ureter at the pelvic brim. In a recent study in Melbourne (Carey et al 1989), 8 cases were recognized at one large obstetric hospital in 1981–1986, whereas only 1 case had been recognized over the preceding 10 years.

Ureteral stents (Goldfarb et al 1989) and percutaneous ureterostomy (Carey et al 1989) have been used to treat ureteric obstruction during pregnancy (Hedegaard & Wallace 1987, Quinn et al 1988). Ureteral stents may be complicated by encrustation of the stent, infection and stone formation (Abber & Kahn 1983, Spirnak & Resnick 1985, Goldfarb et al 1989).

REFERENCES

Abber J C, Kahn R J 1983 Pyelonephritis from severe encrustation on silicone ureteral stents: management. Journal of Urology 130: 763–764

Anderson G W, Rice G G, Harris B A 1949 Pregnancy and labour complicated by pelvic ectopic kidney anomalies. Obstetrical and Gynecological Survey 4: 737–773

Carey M P, Ihle B U, Woodward C S et al 1989 Ureteric obstruction by the gravid uterus. Australian and New Zealand Journal of Obstetrics and Gynaecology 29: 308–313

Eisendrath D N, Rolnick H C 1938 Urology. Lippincott, Philadelphia

Goldfarb R A, Neerhut G J, Lederer E 1989 Management of acute hydronephrosis of pregnancy by ureteral stenting: risk of stone formation. Journal of Urology 141: 921–922

Hedegaard C K, Wallace D 1987 Percutaneous nephrostomy: current indications and potential uses in obstetrics and gynaecology. Literature review and report of a case. Obstetrical and Gynecological Survey 42: 671–675

Hinwood D, Mashire A R 1991 Percutaneous nephrostomy to relieve renal tract obstruction in pregnancy. British Journal of Radiology 64: 976

Killam A, Grillo D, Summerson D J 1967 Pregnancy and delivery after ureterosigmoidoscopy. American Journal of Obstetric Gynecology 97: 278–279

Kock N G, Nilson A E, Norlen L et al 1978 Urinary diversion by a continent ileum reservoir. Scandinavian Journal of Urology and Nephrology, Supplementum 49:23–31

Laverson P L, Hankins G D V, Quirk Jr J G 1984 Ureteral obstruction during pregnancy. Journal of Urology 131: 327–329

Lewis G J, Chatterjee S P, Rowse A D 1985 Acute renal failure presenting in pregnancy secondary to idiopathic hydronephrosis. British Medical Journal 290: 1250–1251

Lowsley O S, Menning J H 1944 Pelvic single kidney. Journal of Urology 51: 117

Muller-Suur R, Tyden O 1985 Evaluation of hydronephrosis in pregnancy using ultrasound and renography. Scandavian Journal of Urology and Nephrology 19: 267–273

Quinn A D, Kusuda L, Amar A D et al 1988 Percutaneous nephrostomy for treatment of hydronephrosis of pregnancy. Journal of Urology 139: 1037–1038

Spirnak J P, Resnick M I 1985 Stone formation as a complication of indwelling ureteral stents: a report of 5 cases. Journal of Urology 134: 349–351

Twickler D, Little B B, Satin A J et al 1991 Renal pelvicalyceal dilation in antepartum pyelonephritis: ultrasonographic findings. American Journal of Obstetrics and Gynecology 65: 1115–1119

Vordermark J S, Deshon G E, Agee R E 1990 Management of pregnancy after major urinary reconstruction. Obstetrics and Gynecology 75: 564–567

6.5 REFLUX NEPHROPATHY AND OTHER TUBULAR INTERSTITIAL DISEASES DURING PREGNANCY

Reflux nephropathy is predominantly a disease of girls and young women. In those who progress, the mean age at which end stage renal failure occurs in women with reflux nephropathy in our department is 33 years, well within the child bearing period. For this reason and because this is a common disease, reflux nephropathy assumes particular importance in relation to pregnancy. Both pregnancy and reflux nephropathy are predisposing factors in urinary tract infection.

6.5.1 Reflux nephropathy, vesicoureteric reflux and bacteriuria

In a consecutive study of 4000 pregnant women, bacteriuria was detected in 6%, and 134 of these women were investigated after pregnancy for underlying renal lesions. As shown in Table 6.1.1–3, 50% of these women showed radiological abnormalities, the most frequent being evidence of focal or diffuse parenchymal scars, characteristic of those described in reflux nephropathy (Hodson 1972). Based on the population of 4000 women studied, this finding suggested that about 1.0% of women in Victoria have this type of parenchymal scarring. It is certainly one of the more frequent renal lesions encountered both in women with bacteriuria and in those with hypertension in pregnancy.

In a study in Wales, vesicoureteric reflux and/or parenchymal scarring was found in 59% of women who had had bacteriuria in pregnancy and in whom bacteriuria was still present 4–6 months post partum. In those women whose urine was sterile 4–6 months post partum but in whom bacteriuria had been present in pregnancy, 13% had reflux nephropathy or vesicoureteric reflux (Williams et al 1968). In a further study in which women who had had childhood urinary tract infection were followed through pregnancy, 47% of women with renal scarring and 27% with no scarring developed bacteriuria in pregnancy compared with only 1–2% of controls (Martinell et al 1990); 6 of the 100 women with bacteriuria developed acute pyelonephritis and 4 of these had underlying radiological abnormalities.

Correction of vesicoureteric reflux does not seem to protect women from pregnancy complications. Austenfeld & Snow (1988) followed up 30 women who had had reimplantation of ureters for primary vesicoureteric reflux in childhood; 17 (57%) of women had urinary tract infection in pregnancy which was acute pyelonephritis in 5, and complete obstruction of the ureter at the vesicoureteric junction occurred during pregnancy in 1. This risk of reimplantation of the ureter has also been observed by Ransley (1983).

All four of these studies demonstrate a very close association between reflux nephropathy and urinary tract infection in pregnancy, and we strongly agree with Williams et al (1968) that pregnant women who have had bacteriuria, particularly those in whom urinary tract infection persists or where there has been difficulty in eradicating the infection and those who develop acute pyelonephritis, should be investigated after pregnancy for reflux nephropathy.

It is of interest that 11 of 21 patients with vesicoureteric reflux persisting to adulthood had no overt parenchymal scarring to indicate the presence of parenchymal renal disease (Williams et al 1968). This indicates that the prevalence of vesicoureteric reflux with or without overt radiological scarring may be double that estimated on the basis of our bacteriuria study in 1965 and may be as high as 2%. In addition to women with overt radiological scars, we see a significant proportion of women presenting with proteinuria in pregnancy in whom the biopsy is suggestive of reflux nephropathy but there are no overt radiographic scars (Kincaid-Smith 1984). Because these women frequently show lateral displacement of the ureteric orifice in the bladder (Kincaid-Smith 1991), we believe they represent another large group of patients with reflux nephropathy which commonly is unrecognized at this time.

Complications of pregnancy in women with vesicoureteric reflux or reflux nephropathy

In our study of 345 pregnancies in 137 women with reflux nephropathy, fetal loss occurred in 14% of pregnancies and prematurity in 3% with an overall rate of fetal complications of 14% (Table 6.5.1–1).

Table 6.5.1–1   Fetal complications in 345 pregnancies (from Beckes et al 1991, with permission)

	No.	Proportion of pregnancies (%)
Fetal loss	48	14
Miscarriage (after 12 weeks' pregnancy)	36	10
Fetal death in utero	6	2
Therapeutic abortion	6	2
Prematurity	12	3
Total fetal complications	50	17

Table 6.5.1–2   Fetal outcome in women with reflux nephropathy and impaired renal function at conception or early in pregnancy (from Jungers et al 1987, with permission)

Plasma creatinine (mmol/l)	No. of pregnancies	Fetal deaths
0.135–0.195	13	7 (53%)
0.20 –0.50	6	5 (83%)
Total	19	12 (63%)

The only other series of cases which included significant patient numbers are those of Jungers et al (1987), who reported on 254 pregnancies in 104 women, and of Arze et al (1982), who reported on 173 pregnancies in 79 women. In both these series the fetal loss rate was similar to our own (12.6% and 19%). These findings substantiate our view that the 10% fetal loss which we observed in women with bacteriuria reflected, in part, the high percentage of patients with lesions of reflux nephropathy (Kincaid-Smith & Bullen 1965).

Fetal loss in reflux nephropathy is clearly related to renal function. Patients with a plasma creatinine above 0.11 mmol/l showed a 24% fetal loss compared with 9% in those with normal function ($P<0.001$) (Kincaid-Smith & Fairley 1987, Becker et al 1991). Jungers' findings in this

Table 6.5.1–3   Maternal complications in 345 pregnancies (from Becker et al 1991, with permission)

	No.	Proportion of pregnancies (%)
Uncomplicated	150	43
Complicated	195	57
Urinary tract infection	70	20
(Acute pyelonephritis)	(19)	(6)
Preeclampsia	59	17
Hypertension or Proteinuria or Oedema	30	9
Deterioration in renal function	13	4
Haematuria	2	1
Stones	3	1

regard (Table 6.5.1–2) are in agreement with ours.

Urinary tract infection occurred more frequently in women with a normal plasma creatinine level,

Table 6.5.1–4   Complications associated with pregnancy in women with normal and impaired renal function (from Becker et al 1991, with permission)

	Plasma creatinine before pregnancy			
	≤0.11 mmol/l 102 women 238 pregnancies	>0.11 mmol/l 23 women 52 pregnancies	RR*	P
Uncomplicated	120 (50%)	8 (15%)		
Complicated	118	44	5.6	<0.001
Urinary tract infection	61 (25%)	6 (12%)	0.4	<0.05
Preeclampsia	32 (13%)	15 (30%)	2.6	<0.025
Hypertension or Proteinuria or Oedema	23 (10%)	3 (6%)		NS
Deterioration in renal function	4 (2%)	9 (18%)	12.2	<0.001
Fetal loss	20 (8%)	9 (18%)	2.3	<0.05

*RR, relative risk associated with impaired renal function.

but all other complications of pregnancy were more frequent in women with a plasma creatinine above 0.11 mmol/l (Table 6.5.1–4)

Preeclampsia was more frequent in women with bilateral renal scarring, occurring in 24% of these women compared with 7% of those with unilateral parenchymal scars (P<0.001).

Women who developed preeclampsia had significantly smaller overall renal size than those who did not (P<0.001) (Becker et al 1991).

Effect of pregnancy on the natural history of reflux nephropathy

Deterioration in renal function was more likely to occur if plasma creatinine was elevated. Only 4 of 238 pregnancies undertaken when renal function was normal were associated with deterioration in renal function compared with deterioration in 9 of 52 pregnancies undertaken when renal function was impaired (P<0.001) (Becker et al 1991). In 6 women with an initial plasma creatinine of 0.2–0.4 mmol/l the rate of decline in renal function was much more rapid than that in women

with the same level of renal impairment who did not become pregnant (Becker et al 1986).

Similar results were obtained by Jungers et al (1987); 4 of 14 women with a plasma creatinine between 0.135 and 0.49 mmol/l showed an accelerated course to end stage renal failure.

Biopsies were carried out in some of our patients with reflux nephropathy in whom deterioration in renal function occurred during pregnancy. These showed fibrin thrombi in glomerular capillaries, suggesting that this change may cause accelerated progression to renal failure (Kincaid-Smith & Fairley 1987).

Because of these observations, and because plasma exchange lowers fibrinogen levels, we have used plasma exchange during pregnancy in the hope of avoiding the inevitable deterioration in renal function observed in untreated patients with a plasma creatinine above 0.2 mmol/l. Figure 6.5.1–1 illustrates the course in a woman with reflux nephropathy treated by plasma exchange. This woman, and another with similar renal function, had a successful pregnancy and in neither was subsequent deterioration in renal function observed over a period of 5 years. In a

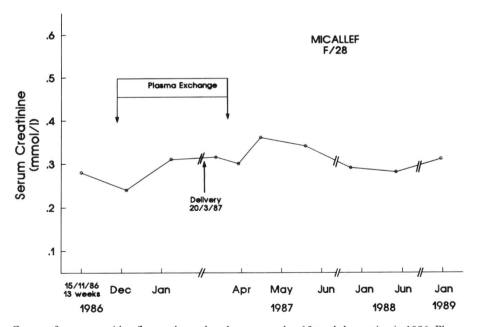

Fig. 6.5.1–1   Course of a women with reflux nephropathy who presented at 13 weeks' gestation in 1986. Plasma exchange during pregnancy and for 3 months after pregnancy maintained stable renal function. Renal function remains stable 5 years after delivery. This course contrasts with the renal course in women with reflux nephropathy and impaired renal function which is marked by rapid deterioration to end stage renal failure.

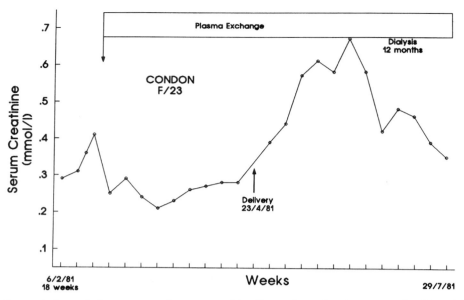

Fig. 6.5.1–2   Course during and after pregnancy in a woman with reflux nephropathy who presented at 18 weeks' gestation with a serum creatinine of 0.3 mmol/l. The serum creatinine improved following plasma exchange and stabilized for several weeks. Early delivery because of deteriorating function did not halt the deterioration which continued for 6 weeks after delivery. Over the subsequent 6 weeks the serum creatinine fell to 0.37 mmol/l but after cessation of plasma exchange it declined again and dialysis was commenced 12 months after delivery.

third patient with a serum creatinine of just below 0.3 mmol/l (Fig. 6.5.1–2), although plasma exchange through pregnancy virtually improved renal function, it subsequently declined despite early delivery and deterioration continued to the postdelivery period. Continuation of plasma exchange slowly reversed this trend and 3 months after delivery the level had returned almost to the level at presentation. In spite of this recovery the patient subsequently deteriorated and required dialysis 12 months after delivery.

Reflux nephropathy is a familial disease and pregnancy in women with reflux nephropathy also represents an ideal opportunity for the diagnosis of vesicoureteric reflux in the infant. Dilatation of the renal pelvis in the fetus is one method of detecting vesicoureteric reflux in the infant (Najmaldin et al 1990, Gordon et al 1990). Another non invasive ultrasound technique which promises to provide a good screening test for vesicoureteric reflux in the newborn is the so-called 'jet study'. In this technique a colour doppler image of the jets of urine entering the

bladder permit the visualization of the site of the vesicoureteric orifice. Refluxing ureters are lateral in position (Marshall et al 1990).

6.5.2   Other tubular interstitial diseases

There is surprisingly little documentation of the course of other tubular interstitial diseases in pregnancy.

The more common tubular interstitial diseases such as analgesic nephropathy and urate nephropathy tend to affect women beyond the child bearing years.

In their 1980 analysis, Katz et al (1980) reported on 26 pregnancies in 21 women with 'interstitial nephritis'. This appeared to be a group with a relatively good prognosis for both mother and fetus. Our studies suggest that by far the most frequent tubular interstitial lesion encountered on biopsy in young women is reflux nephropathy, but the nature of the underlying lesion in the cases of Katz et al (1980) is not documented.

REFERENCES

Arze R S, Ramos J M, Owen J A et al 1982 The natural history of chronic pyelonephritis in the adult. Quarterly Journal of Medicine 51: 396–410

Austenfeld M S, Snow B W 1988 Complications of pregnancy in women after reimplantation for vesicoureteral reflux. Journal of Urology 140: 1103–1106

Becker G J, Ihle B U, Fairley K F, Bastos M, Kincaid-Smith P 1986 Effect of pregnancy on moderate renal failure in reflux nephropathy. British Medical Journal 292: 796–798

Becker G J, El-Khatib M, Kincaid-Smith P 1991 Pregnancy related complications in women with reflux nephropathy. Clinical Nephrology in press

Gordon A C, Thomas D F M, Arthur R J, Irving H C, Smith SEW 1990 Parentally diagnosed reflux: a follow-study. British Journal of Urology 65: 407–412

Hodson C J 1972 Radiology of the Kidney. In: Sir Douglas Black (ed) Renal Disease. Blackwell Scientific Publications, Oxford. 3rd edition, Chapter 8, pp 213–249

Jungers P, Houillier P, Forget D 1987 Reflux nephropathy and pregnancy. Baillieres Clinical Obstetrics and Gynaecology 1:955–969

Katz A I, Davison J M, Hayslett J P, Singson E, Lindheimer M D 1980 Pregnancy in women with kidney disease. Kidney International 18: 192–206

Kincaid-Smith P 1984 Diffuse parenchymal lesions in reflux nephropathy and the possibility of making a renal biopsy diagnosis in reflux nephropathy In: C J Hodson, R H Heptinstall, J Winberg (eds) Reflux nephropathy update 1983. Contributions to nephrology. Karger, Basel, vol 39: pp 111–115

Kincaid-Smith P 1991 Reflux nephropathy without overt radiological lesions. In: Bailey R R (ed) Proceedings, 2nd CJ Hodson Symposium. Sandoz, Christchurch

Kincaid-Smith P, Bullen M 1965 Bacteriuria in pregnancy. Lancet 1: 395–399

Kincaid-Smith P, Fairley K F 1987 Renal disease in pregnancy. Three controversial areas: mesangial IgA nephropathy, focal glomerular sclerosis (focal and segmental hyalinosis and sclerosis), and reflux nephropathy. American Journal of Kidney Diseases 9: 328–333

Marshall J L, Johnson N D, De Campo M P 1990 Vesicoureteric reflux in children: prediction with colour doppler imaging — work in progress 1. Radiology 175: 355–358

Martinell J, Jodal U, Lidin-Janson G 1990 Pregnancies in women with and without renal scarring after urinary infections in childhood. British Medical Journal 300: 840–844

Najmaldin A, Burge D M, Atwell J D 1990 Paediatric urology. Fetal vesicoureteric reflux. British Journal of Urology 65: 403–406

Ransley P G 1983 Personal communication

Williams G L, Davies D K L, Evans K T 1968 Vesicoureteric reflux in patients with bacteriuria in pregnancy. Lancet 2: 1202–1205

6.6 IDIOPATHIC GLOMERULONEPHRITIS

We have recently analysed our experience in pregnancy in the different histological subtypes of glomerulonephritis; the methodology in each group has been similar and is set out in this section.

Because in some subgroups such as mesangial proliferative glomerulonephritis, we were dependent upon fluorescent or immunoperoxidase staining of deposits in order to place a biopsy in a particular category, some of these analyses, as for example mesangial IgA glomerulonephritis, only date back to 1971 which was the year in which we first had reliable routine identification of immunoglobulins in glomeruli. In other histological subgroups which could be clearly identified by light or electron microscopy, we included all patients back to 1959 when our prospective collection of data on patients with renal disease in pregnancy commenced.

The methods used in the analysis were similar in the different histological groups. The biopsy processing techniques are described elsewhere (Kincaid-Smith et al 1985)

Fetal outcome

For each pregnancy, including those resulting in first trimester fetal loss, the duration of gestation and fetal outcome were recorded. Indications for therapeutic abortion or induction of premature labour were noted.

Prematurity was defined as gestation of between 32 and 36 weeks. Severe prematurity was defined as prior to 32 weeks.

Birth weights were available for the majority of infants, and infants were classified as small for gestational age if their birth weights fell below the tenth percentile for the Australian population.

Maternal outcome

The blood pressure, 24-h urine protein, plasma creatinine and urea were recorded in each trimester and for 6 months after the pregnancy. Where available, prepregnancy values were also recorded.

The past obstetric history and any treatment received during pregnancy were recorded.

Impaired renal function was defined as a plasma creatinine >0.11 mmol/l or plasma urea >8.3 mmol/l prior to, or during, pregnancy or as $\geqslant$50% increase in these values during pregnancy.

Proteinuria was defined as $\geqslant 0.15$ g/24 h prior to pregnancy and $\geqslant 0.3$ g/24 h during pregnancy. Increased proteinuria during pregnancy was defined as an increase of $\geqslant 0.2$ g/24 h if initial excretion was <0.5 g/24 h or as a doubling of the 24 h excretion if initial values exceed 0.5 g/24 h. Nephrotic range proteinuria was defined as >5 g protein in 24 h. Prior to pregnancy hypertension was defined as $\geqslant 95$ mmHg, or as a requirement for antihypertensive medication, and during pregnancy as a diastolic blood pressure of 90 mmHg or an increase of $\geqslant 15$ mmHg. Hypertension was considered to be 'severe' in pregnancy if diastolic blood pressure was $\geqslant 110$ mmHg and to have occurred 'early' if it developed prior to 32 weeks' gestation. An exacerbation of preexisting hypertension during pregnancy was defined as a diastolic blood pressure of $\geqslant 90$ mmHg despite continued antihypertensive treatment.

Reversibility was defined as a complete resolution of impaired renal function or hypertension (on no treatment) within 6 months postpartum. Reversibility of proteinuria was defined as a halving in maximal 24 h protein excretion if >0.5 g/24 h or as a reduction by >0.2 g/24 h if maximal excretion was <0.5 g/24 h.

Statistical analysis was done using the χ^2 test.

An overview of the results of pregnancy in women with glomerulonephritis is considered in 6.6.4 at the end of the discussion of the details in the separate morphological categories of glomerulonephritis.

For details of the morphological classification of glomerulonephritis used in these studies readers are referred to Kincaid-Smith & Whitworth (1987).

REFERENCES

Kincaid-Smith P, Whitworth J A (eds) 1987 The kidney, 2nd edn. Blackwell Scientific, Oxford
Kincaid-Smith P, Dowling J P, Mathews D C (eds) 1985 Atlas of glomerular disease. Morphological and clinical correlation. Adis Health Science Press

6.6.1 Pregnancy in women with diffuse non-lgA mesangial proliferative glomerulonephritis including thin basement membrane disease

Apart from our own publication (Packham et al 1988) there is very little documentation of the fetal or maternal outcome of pregnancy in women with diffuse mesangial proliferative glomerulonephritis without associated mesangial IgA deposits.

Because this is one of the most frequent conditions which we encounter, we had available the records of 168 pregnancies in 91 women in this histological subgroup of glomerulonephritis.

Most women with non-IgA diffuse mesangial proliferative glomerulonephritis present with isolated microscopic haematuria (Kincaid-Smith et al 1991), and many units would not carry out a renal biopsy in such patients. The degree of microscopic haematuria is often quite heavy in such patients, frequently above 200 000 per ml. The other likely diagnosis in patients with isolated microscopic haematuria is mesangial IgA glomerulonephritis (Kincaid-Smith et al 1991) and because continuing microscopic haematuria of this degree has the strongest predictive value for progression in mesangial IgA glomerulonephritis (Nicholls et al 1984) we have always had a policy of carrying out biopsies in patients with isolated microscopic haematuria of this degree. The dearth of data from other centres about pregnancy in patients with this histological subgroup may well relate to biopsy policy.

Abe et al (1985) reported on 35 pregnancies in 25 women with non-IgA diffuse mesangial proliferative glomerulonephritis and, as some centres in Japan do carry out biopsies in patients with isolated microscopic haematuria, these patients may well represent a similar group to ours. Katz et al (1980) included 3 pregnancies in 26 women with diffuse proliferative glomerulonephritis. As these women were collected from three units over a period prior to 1980, it seems likely that these patients had other indications for renal biopsy such as the nephrotic syndrome or proteinuria, and they may represent a more severe group of patients because of prevailing policies at that time concerning indications for renal biopsy in the United States and the United Kingdom would not normally have included the indication of isolated microscopic haematuria.

The 91 women were supervised jointly by members of the nephrology department at the Royal Melbourne Hospital and the obstetric staff of the Royal Women's Hospital. They presented between 1968 and 1986.

The histological lesion

The glomerular lesions of diffuse mesangial proliferative glomerulonephritis without mesangial IgA deposits are very similar in different cases. The glomeruli are usually increased in size. By definition they show a diffuse increase in mesangial cells (Fig. 6.6.1–1) and this is almost invariably accompanied by an increase in mesangial matrix. Mesangial deposits are not seen on Masson stains, and this distinguishes this lesion from that of mesangial IgA glomerulonephritis.

When stained with antisera against immunoglobulins and complement components and fibrin by immunofluorescence or immunoperoxidase microscopy, there maybe no positive staining. Commonly small amounts of mesangial IgM, C3 and C1q are seen.

Thin basement membrane disease

There is uncertainty at this time as to what proportion of patients with this type of diffuse mesangial proliferative lesions without mesangial IgA deposits show thin basement membranes on electron microscopy. Many of them do, but unfortunately relatively few of the 91 women

included in this study had electron microscopy performed. We now perform electron microscopy in all such cases and the majority show thin basement membranes (Kincaid-Smith et al 1991). The characteristic feature is very striking in some cases (Fig. 6.6.1–2). There remains some uncertainty as to the lower level of normal for the width of the glomerular basement membrane but it is likely that the majority of the 91 women included in this report have thin basement membrane.

The methods of analysis used in this group of patients with glomerulonephritis were the same as those used in other groups as outlined under 6.6. In this group, however, where the basic pattern of lesions in glomeruli are mild, the influence of superimposed lesions such as vessel changes, sclerosed glomeruli and focal and segmental hyalinosis is likely to be more pronounced and these were also analysed.

Table 6.6.1–1 illustrates the foetal outcome in the 108 pregnancies in 91 women. There was one set of twins.

The fetal loss in this series was 20% but, if spontaneous and therapeutic abortions are excluded, there was a fetal loss of 12% after 20 weeks. This is the same percentage of fetal loss as

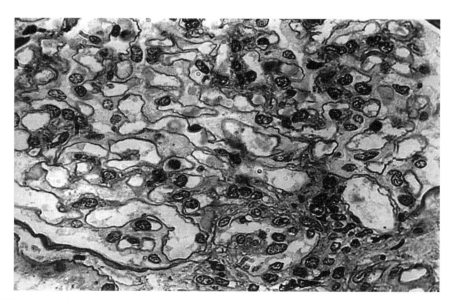

Fig. 6.6.1–1   Diffuse mesangial proliferative glomerulonephritis without mesangial IgA deposits showing clear cut proliferation of mesangial cells and some increase in mesangial matrix.

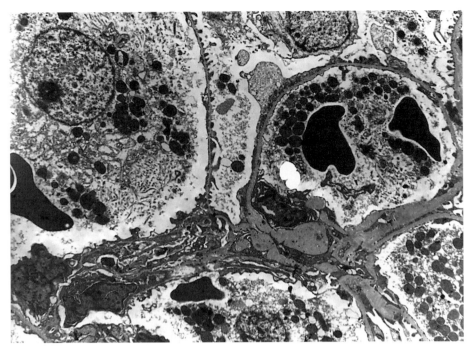

Fig. 6.6.1–2 Electron micrograph illustrating the features of thin basement membrane disease. The basement membranes of glomerular capillaries show marked thinning.

that recorded by Abe et al (1985) in 35 pregnancies in 23 women with non-IgA diffuse proliferative glomerulonephritis. Katz et al (1980) included data on 33 pregnancies in 26 women with 'diffuse glomerulonephritis' and recorded

Table 6.6.1–1 Outcome of 169 fetuses in 168 pregnancies in 91 women with non-IgA mesangial proliferative glomerulonephritis (from Packham et al 1988, with permission)

Fetal outcome	No. of fetuses	%
Fetal loss		
Therapeutic abortions	2	1
Spontaneous abortions	11	7
Stillbirths	12	7
Neonatal deaths	8	5
Total fetal loss	33	20
Live infants		
Prematurity		
≤32 weeks' gestation	12	7
32–37 weeks' gestation	19	11
Term		
>37 weeks' gestation	105	62
Total live infants	136	80

fetal loss after the first trimester in 18% of cases but, as discussed above, it is likely that these cases represented a more severe group who may well have had biopsy indications including the nephrotic syndrome or proteinuria. Table 6.6.1–1 also shows that 18% of pregnancies resulted in premature delivery which was severe in 12 cases (7%). Figure 6.6.1–3 shows the birth weight of 109 fetuses for whom results were available; 15 infants (14%) were small for gestational age, which is not significantly different from the normal population. Considering the mild glomerular lesions, in most cases with diffuse mesangial proliferative glomerulonephritis, and the generally benign prognosis in such patients, it is perhaps surprising that the fetal loss in both our series and Abe's series was so high. The fetal loss in Victoria in 1980 was 1.37% and thus a 12% fetal loss appears high for a relatively benign renal condition. All but 6% of patients presented to us with complications of pregnancy and this may well explain the relatively high fetal loss because one would anticipate a worse prognosis in

INTRAUTERINE GROWTH CHART

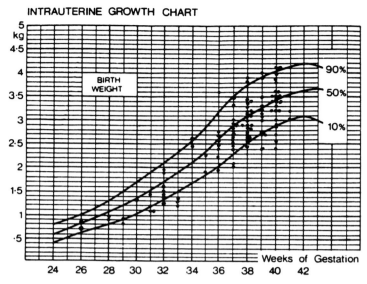

Fig. 6.6.1–3   Birth weights of 109 fetuses of mothers with non-IgA mesangial proliferative glomerulonephritis.

patients who present with pregnancy related complications (Packham et al 1989).

Looking for other reasons why this generally benign renal lesion might be associated with a fetal loss rate of 12%, we analysed other histological features which could contribute to this outcome. On analysing the effect of sclerosed glomeruli and superimposed lesions of focal and segmental hyalinosis on the biopsy specimen, 27 pregnancies in 15 women were found to be associated with sclerosis of over 10% of glomeruli on biopsy, and 30 pregnancies in 13 women showed superimposed focal and segmental hyalinosis. Although the fetal outcome tended to be worse in pregnancies of women who showed these additional features, on biopsy the differences between those without these superimposed lesions were not significant (Packham et al 1988).

Another histological feature which did have an impact on the outcome of pregnancy was the presence of severe vessel lesions on renal biopsy. The presence of severe vessel lesions on renal biopsy and the influence on the outcome of pregnancy is shown in Table 6.6.1–2. Total fetal loss was very high in women with severe vessel lesions (36%), and significantly worse than the outcome in women whose biopsies did not show severe vessel lesions ($P<0.0005$). The incidence of prematurity was also much higher in women

with severe vessel lesions (32%) compared with those whose biopsies did not show severe vessel lesions (12%) ($P<0.005$).

The maternal outcome in 91 women (168 pregnancies) is shown in Table 6.6.1–3. As might be expected in this relatively mild form of glomerulonephritis the frequency of irreversible impairment of renal function, hypertension and proteinuria following pregnancy is not as high in this histological group as in some other forms of glomerulonephritis reported in 6.6.2–6.6.7.

Reversible decline in renal function occurred in 3% of cases, reversible hypertension in 33% and reversible increases in proteinuria in 52% of cases.

The influence of severe vessel lesions on renal biopsy on the maternal outcome is shown in Table 6.6.1–2. Although the number of patients with a more serious outcome was higher for each complication when severe vessel lesions were seen on biopsy, only one — that of early hypertension — was statistically significant ($P<0.005$). With larger numbers it is likely that other features such as impairment of renal function might have become significant. 7 patients whose biopsies showed severe vessel lesions showed a deterioration of renal function during pregnancy compared with only 1 in the group without severe vessel lesions (Table 6.6.1–2).

Table 6.6.1–2   Comparison of pregnancies in patients with and without severe vessel lesions (from Packham et al 1988, with permission)

Outcome	Severe (26 women, 57 pregnancies)		Non-severe (65 women, 111 pregnancies)	
	No. of pregnancies	%	No. of pregnancies	%
Fetal outcome				
Fetal loss	21	36*	12	11
Prematurity	18	32	13	12†
Term	18	21	87	77*
Total Fetuses	57	100	112	100
Maternal outcome				
Impaired renal function	4	7	1	1
Hypertension				
Irreversible	3	5	8	7
Reversible	22	39	33	30
Exacerbation	8	14	6	5
Total	33	58	47	42
Stable	3	5	3	3
Early	21	37†	18	16†
Severe	15	26	15	14
Proteinuria increased	36	63	53	48

*$P<0.0005$, †$P<0.005$.

Where the presence of hypertension prior to pregnancy was considered in terms of its influence on fetal and maternal outcome, although there is an increased fetal loss and higher rate of prematurity in women who were hypertensive before pregnancy, these did not reach statistical significance.

Similarly, although the maternal outcome in women who were hypertensive before pregnancy included a higher rate of hypertension, early hypertension and increased proteinuria, these differences were not statistically significant.

We have previously described and illustrated a case in which a mild diffuse mesangial proliferative lesion demonstrated on biopsy in early pregnancy deteriorated to an unusual mesangiocapillary form of glomerulonephritis during pregnancy (Fairley et al 1973, Kincaid-Smith 1975). This unusual biopsy change persisted on a renal biopsy taken 10 years later. This type of change is obviously both unusual and rare but, in the case of the patient concerned, clearly represented a significant histological deterioration.

In Abe's series (1985), which is the only one with sufficient numbers to warrant comparison with our patients, those patients who were diagnosed prior to pregnancy did better than those presenting during pregnancy. Patients diagnosed prior to pregnancy are a selected group because those with more severe clinical or histological features might be advised against pregnancy.

Table 6.6.1–3   Maternal outcome of 168 pregnancies in 91 women with non-IgA mesangial proliferative glomerulonephritis (from Packham et al 1988, with permission)

Maternal outcome	No. of pregnancies	%
Impaired renal function		
Irreversible	0	0
Reversible	5	3
Total	5	3
Hypertension		
Irreversible	11	7
Reversible	55	33
Exacerbation	14	8
Total	88	48
Stable	6	4
Proteinuria		
Irreversible increase	2	1
Reversible increase	87	52
Total	89	53
Stable	13	8

Patients diagnosed before pregnancy also receive more careful supervision during pregnancy Only 6% of our patients were diagnosed before pregnancy in this histological subgroup, the majority presented during pregnancy with complications of pregnancy.

Abe et al (1985) were unable to demonstrate any difference in fetal or maternal outcome between their patients with IgA and non-IgA diffuse mesangial proliferative glomerulonephritis. We, on the other hand, have demonstrated higher fetal loss, impairment of renal function, hypertension and increase proteinuria in mesangial IgA glomerulonephritis than in non-IgA mesangial proliferative glomerulonephritis (see 6.6.2).

Overall, the results in pregnancy in patients with diffuse non-IgA mesangial proliferative glomerulonephritis are, in our hands, rather better than those in other forms of glomerulonephritis. This is in keeping with the generally benign course of this form of glomerulonephritis and the fact that it includes the benign inherited condition, thin basement membrane disease, which carries a good long term prognosis.

In women in this subgroup of glomerulonephritis it is worth checking the infant's urine for microscopic haematuria. In the infants of women with thin basement membrane disease, urine abnormalities may be apparent at a very early age, and half the infants born to women with thin basement membrane disease have haematuria.

REFERENCES

Abe S, Amagasaki Y, Konishi K et al 1985 The influence of antecedent renal disease on pregnancy. American Journal of Obstetrics and Gynecology 153: 508–514

Fairley K F, Whitworth J A, Kincaid-Smith P 1973 Glomerulonephritis and pregnancy. In: P Kincaid-Smith, T H Mathew, E L Becker (eds) Glomerulonephritis. Wiley, New York, p 997

Katz A L, Davison J M, Hayslett J P et al 1980 Pregnancy in women with kidney disease. Kidney International 18: 192

Kincaid-Smith P (ed) 1975 The kidney — a clinicopathological study. Blackwell Scientific, Oxford

Kincaid-Smith P, Owen J, Hewitson T 1991 Unexplained haematuria. British Medical Journal 302: 177–178

Nicholls K M, Fairley K F, Dowling J P et al 1984 The clinical course of mesangial IgA nephropathy. Quarterly Journal of Medicine 53: 227–250

Packham D K, North R A, Fairley K F et al 1988 Pregnancy in women with diffuse mesangial proliferative glomerulonephritis. Clinical Nephrology 29: 193–198

Packham D K, North R A, Fairley K F et al 1989 Primary glomerulonephritis and pregnancy. Quarterly Journal of Medicine (New Series 71) 266: 537–553

6.6.2 Mesangial IgA glomerulonephritis

Our experience of pregnancy in patients with mesangial IgA glomerulonephritis has been recorded in a number of previous publications (Packham et al 1988a, b, Kincaid-Smith et al 1980, Kincaid-Smith & Fairley 1987, Whitworth et al 1982).

We have documented the results of 116 pregnancies in 79 women with mesangial IgA glomerulonephritis seen between 1971 and 1986. We did not include patients seen prior to 1971 because that was the first year in which identification of IgA deposits in the mesangium was routinely available on renal biopsy specimens. Patients with clinical features suggesting Henoch–Schönlein syndrome are also excluded. The date of the renal biopsy antedated the pregnancy in only 4 patients (6%) so that 25 (36%) presented to us during pregnancy, and the biopsy, confirming the diagnosis, was carried out after the pregnancy (within 12 months) in 41 (58%).

The histological lesion of mesangial IgA glomerulonephritis is illustrated by Masson staining in Figure 6.6.2–1. It may be possible to be almost sure of the diagnosis using Masson stains because of the presence of large red staining paramesangial deposits which are characteristic. It is important, however, to confirm the diagnosis using specific fluorescein or immunoperoxidase labelling of the IgA deposits in the mesangium.

The data collected in these patients were as set out in 6.6 and are similar to that for other categories in glomerulonephritis.

We have shown that in mesangial IgA glomerulonephritis the histological features influence the outcome during pregnancy (Packham et al 1988a); 27 (38%) patients showed a diffuse mesangial proliferative lesion on renal biopsy, 30 (43%) had superimposed focal and segmental proliferative lesion.

The results are first analysed for the whole group of patients and subsequently the influence of the histological features is considered.

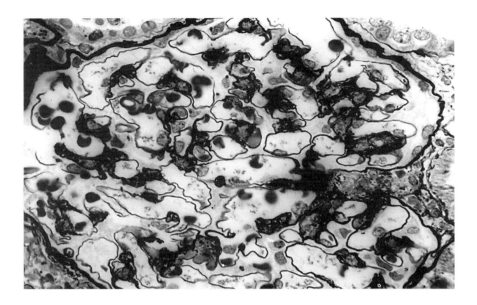

Fig. 6.6.2–1

The fetal outcome is summarized in Table 6.6.2–1. The fetal loss rate was high at 30% and if therapeutic abortions are excluded it remains high at 26%. Almost all the stillbirths and neonatal deaths occurred in pregnancies complicated by early hypertension and increased proteinuria; 26% of infants were born prematurely and 4% were severely premature (before 32 weeks' gestation).

Table 6.6.2–1   Outcome of 118 fetuses and 116* pregnancies in 70 women with IgA glomerulonephritis (from Packham et al 1988b, with permission)

Fetal outcome	No. of fetuses	%
Fetal loss		
Therapeutic abortions	6	5
Spontaneous abortions	4	3
Stillbirths	16*	14
Neonatal deaths	9	8
Total fetal loss	35	30
Live infants		
Prematurity		
<32 weeks' gestation	5	4
32–37 weeks' gestation	26	22
Term		
≥37 weeks' gestation	52	44
Total live births	83	70

*Includes two sets of twins.

Birth weights, which were available for 72 infants, are shown in Figure 6.6.2–2; 7 infants (10%) were small for gestational age.

These results do not differ greatly from the only other large study of the outcome of pregnancy in patients with mesangial IgA glomerulonephritis. Jungers et al published data on 69 pregnancies in 34 women and recorded a 20% fetal loss (Jungers et al 1986).

Abe et al (1985), in a much smaller study, reported a 13% fetal loss excluding therapeutic abortions. This compares with our fetal loss rate of 22% when therapeutic abortions are excluded. The higher perinatal mortality in our study is likely to reflect the fact that our unit is a tertiary referral centre for renal complications related to pregnancy and that 36% of our patients presented in pregnancy with complications — a factor which automatically selects a more serious group of cases. Table 6.6.2–2 shows that the rate of fetal loss, where the patient is referred for a pregnancy related complication, is double that in pregnancies undertaken after the diagnosis is known, 36% compared with 16%, and this could well influence our overall results.

The maternal outcome in our patients with mesangial IgA glomerulonephritis is summarized

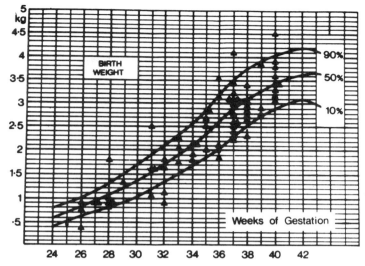

Fig. 6.6.2–2   Birth weight at gestation of 72 infants born to mothers with mesangial IgA glomerulonephritis.

in Table 6.6.2–3. Renal function declined during pregnancy in 30 (26%) pregnancies. In all but 2 renal function returned to the previous level within 6 months of pregnancy.

Only 1 patient had impaired renal function in early pregnancy. She presented at 13 weeks with a serum creatinine of 0.24 mmol/l. Renal biopsy showed advanced lesions with both focal and segmental hyalinosis and sclerosis in addition to active crescents on biopsy. She suffered an antepartum haemorrhage and delivery of a premature infant at 26 weeks; the infant survived 6 days. Following delivery she developed severe hypertension associated with rapid deterioration in renal function and required dialysis within months.

Table 6.6.2–2   Comparison of pregnancies undertaken pre and post diagnosis (from Packham et al 1988b with permission)

Fetal outcome	Pre diagnosis 43 women 79 pregnancies 81 fetuses		Post diagnosis 27 women 37 pregnancies 37 fetuses	
	No. of fetuses	%	No. of fetuses	%
Fetal loss				
Therapeutic abortions	3	4	3	8
Spontaneous abortions	3	4	1	3
Stillbirths	15	19	1	3
Neonatal deaths	8	10	1	3
Total fetal loss	29	36	6	16
Live infants				
Prematurity				
<32 weeks' gestation	1	1	4	11
32–37 weeks' gestation	22	27	4	11
Term				
≥37 weeks' gestation	29	36	23	62
Total live infants	52	64	31	84

Table 6.6.2–3   Maternal outcome of 116 pregnancies in 70 women with IgA nephropathy (from Packham 1988b, with permission)

Maternal outcome	No. of pregnancies	%
Impaired renal function		
Irreversible	2	2
Reversible	28	24
Total	30	26
Hypertension		
Irreversible	15	13
Reversible	37	32
Exacerbation	9	8
Total	61	52
Stable	9	8
Proteinuria		
Irreversible increase	12	10
Reversible increase	62	53
Total	74	63
Stable	19	16

The second patient, who deteriorated during pregnancy, had normal renal function before pregnancy, became nephrotic and showed active crescents on biopsy. Massive proteinuria (12 g/ 24 h) followed delivery at 34 weeks and the serum creatinine remained elevated after pregnancy. This patient progressed to end stage renal failure over 4 years, an unusually rapid course for a woman presenting with mesangial IgA glomerulonephritis and normal renal function.

Three other patients whose renal function deteriorated for the first time during pregnancy showed some improvement by 6 months postpartum but all subsequently progressed to end stage renal failure in 3, 4 and 7 years, respectively.

De novo hypertension appeared during pregnancy or preexisting hypertension increased during pregnancy in 61 (52%) cases. In 15 (13%) this rise in blood pressure had not reversed by 6 months post partum. In half of the 18 women who had hypertension prior to pregnancy an exacerbation occurred during pregnancy in spite of medication.

Severe hypertension with a diastolic blood pressure over 110 mmHg occurred in 20 (17%) pregnancies, this level of blood pressure being one which is judged to constitute a threat to the mother in terms of complications of hypertension. This degree of hypertension is rarely encountered in women with mesangial IgA glomerulonephritis who are not pregnant (Nicholls et al 1984). Proteinuria was present in 79% of pregnancies and an increase was documented in 74 (63%). This pregnancy related increase in proteinuria had not disappeared 6 months after the pregnancy in 12 (10%). Nephrotic range proteinuria (>5 g/24 h) occurred in 10 women (9%).

While decline in renal function, increasing de novo hypertension and increasing proteinuria were irreversible in only a relatively small percentage of cases, these three parameters are the major risk factors predicting progression in mesangial IgA glomerulonephritis. (Kincaid-Smith & Nicholls 1983, Nicholls et al 1984). The major evidence that pregnancy influences the natural history of glomerulonephritis rests on this observed deterioration in these three clearly defined risk factors for progression (Nicholls et al 1984). An irreversible decline in renal function in 2% of cases, a permanent increase in blood pressure in 13% of cases and an increase in proteinuria in 10% of cases over the short period of a pregnancy cannot be regarded as part of the natural history of mesangial IgA glomerulonephritis, nor can the severe hypertension which developed in 20 patients (Kincaid-Smith & Nicholls 1983, Nicholls et al 1984).

Surian et al (1984), in a study of 29 pregnancies undertaken by 21 women, reported development of hypertension in 20% of cases, and Jungers et al (1986) reported hypertension in 39% of their series of 69 pregnancies in women with mesangial IgA glomerulonephritis. Neither series recorded the blood pressure findings in the same detail as we have been able to document but their findings add some support to ours. Jungers et al (1986) recorded increased proteinuria in 32% of cases and decline renal function in 39%.

Of the Jungers et al (1986) patients with mesangial IgA glomerulonephritis 9% progressed to end stage renal failure within 1 year post partum. Considering the relatively benign course of this disease in women and the very gradual progression to end stage renal failure, which occurs on average over a period of 17 years and in only 10% of women with mesangial IgA glomerulonephritis (Nicholls et al 1984), we would believe that this suggests that Jungers et al's (1986) experience, like ours, supports the view that pregnancy contributed to accelerated progression to end stage renal failure in these patients.

Mesangial IgA glomerulonephritis is a condition in which segmental lesions assume particular significance. A diffuse mesangial proliferative lesion in which segmental lesions do not develop never progresses in our experience. In such patients we have observed stable renal histology, renal function and blood pressure over 30 years. The patients who progress do so by the development of segmental lesions.

A very small number of patients, almost all of whom are men, show a rapidly progressive deterioration in renal function accompanied by destruction of glomeruli by crescents which are present in a high percentage of glomeruli in such cases (Nicholls et al 1985).

Crescents are often observed on biopsies done during pregnancy in women with mesangial IgA glomerulonephritis. Because crescents may occur as part of the natural history of mesangial IgA glomerulonephritis, it is not as easy to attribute crescent formation which occurs during preg-

nancy in such cases to the influence of the pregnancy as it is in, for example, membranous glomerulonephritis in which crescents do not occur outside the context of pregnancy.

One of the histological observations which makes it likely that crescents in glomerulonephritis result from superimposed preeclampsia is their occurrence in close proximity to characteristic subendothelial fibrinoid deposits which are the hallmark of preeclampsia.

Figure 6.6.2–3 illustrates a crescent in close proximity to subendothelial deposits of preeclampsia in a woman with mesangial IgA glomerulonephritis whose renal function deteriorated during pregnancy. Segmental crescents in this patient (Fairley & Packham 1989) were very clearly seen to be present in areas adjacent to typical subendothelial deposits of preeclampsia. We have also reported this proximity of crescents to the typical glomerular lesions of preeclampsia in membranous glomerulonephritis (Fairley et al 1973).

The significance of the lesion of focal and segmental hyalinosis is not as clear cut as that of crescent formation in mesangial IgA glomerulonephritis. Many years ago we recorded the lesion

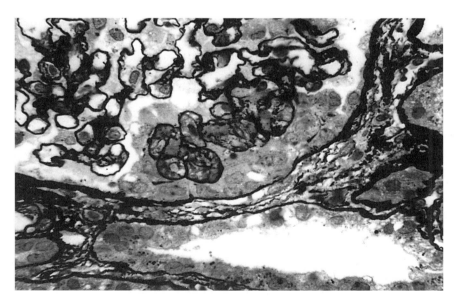

Fig. 6.6.2–3   Glomerulus from a biopsy taken during pregnancy in a women with mesangial IgA glomerulonephritis in whom crescents developed during pregnancy. The crescent formation in the lower right hand quadrant of the glomerulus is strictly confined to an area in the glomerulus where subendothelial deposits typical of preeclampsia are present.

of superimposed focal and segmental hyalinosis in a wide variety of different conditions including pregnancy (Kincaid-Smith 1975). Although focal and segmental hyalinosis is a relatively uncommon lesion in biopsies from women with mesangial IgA glomerulonephritis, it was noted in 8 of 12 biopsies carried out in women in pregnancy or in the early postpartum period (Kincaid-Smith et al 1980, Whitworth et al 1982). This contrasts with the rarity of focal and segmental hyalinosis in biopsies in women with mesangial IgA glomerulonephritis who are not pregnant. When we compared biopsies carried out during pregnancy or in the early postpartum period with biopsies in 67 women which were done at a time remote from pregnancy, we found a highly significant increase in the lesion of focal segmental hyalinosis in pregnancy associated biopsies (Table 6.6.2–4).

Focal and segmental hyalinosis is now regarded as part of the pathology of preeclampsia (Nochy et al 1986, Kida et al 1985, Kincaid-Smith & Fairley 1987, Nagai et al 1991) and its frequency in biopsies which are related in time to a pregnancy (Table 6.6.2–4) may merely represent 'superimposed preeclampsia'.

Because the histological lesions in mesangial IgA glomerulonephritis have a major impact on the prognosis in the individual patient the influence of the histological lesion has been analysed in relation to the outcome of pregnancy (Packham et al 1988a).

The fetal outcome in the different histological subgroups of mesangial IgA glomerulonephritis is shown in Table 6.6.2–5.

Focal and segmental hyalinosis was present as a superimposed lesion in 43% of biopsies, whereas 38% showed diffuse mesangial proliferative glomerulonephritis with no superimposed segmental lesions and only 19% showed superimposed focal and segmental proliferative lesions (usually crescents).

Although both fetal loss (50%) and prematurity (39%) were present in a higher percentage of women with focal and segmental proliferative lesions, the differences did not reach statistical significance in view of the small numbers in the different groups.

The maternal outcome is also summarized in Table 6.6.2–5. The number of patients with impaired renal function was significantly higher in patients with focal and segmental proliferative lesions. An overall 'bad maternal outcome', defined as persisting impairment of renal function, increased proteinuria or development of hypertension, was also significantly higher in the focal and segmental proliferative group.

Focal and segmental proliferative lesions are essentially the lesions associated with crescent formation but patients are still placed in that histological subgroup if the crescents are healed or healing. In 8 patients, active cellular crescents associated with fibrin formation were noted.

Neither the presence of the >10% sclerosed glomeruli nor the presence of active crescents on biopsy affected the fetal or maternal outcome (Table 6.6.2–6).

When the results in pregnancy in women whose biopsies did and did not show severe vessel lesions are compared, the rate of fetal loss is seen to be significantly higher in women whose biopsies showed severe vessel lesions, 54% in this group suffering fetal loss compared with 23% in the other group $P<0.02$) (Table 6.6.2–7).

Abe et al (1985) also reported worse results in pregnancy in women with arteriolar lesions on biopsy, but they included all forms of renal disease in their analysis, not just mesangial IgA glomerulonephritis.

We previously noted this association between severe vessel lesions and outcome of pregnancy. We also demonstrated an increase in vessel lesions during the course of a pregnancy in individual patients (Kincaid-Smith et al 1973).

A particular group of patients in whom severe vessel lesions develop during pregnancy and are

Table 6.6.2–4   Segmental lesions in IgA glomerulonephritis (from Kincaid-Smith & Fairley 1987, with permission)

	Biopsies during pregnancy and early postpartum period	Other biopsies
Focal and segmental hyalinosis	8	6
No focal and segmental hyalinosis	4	61
Total	12	67

$\chi^2 = 21.52$, $P<0.005$.

Table 6.6.2–5 Fetal and maternal outcome of 118 fetuses and 116 pregnancies of 70 women with IgA nephropathy divided into histological groups (from Packham et al 1988a, with permission)

	DMP		FSHS		FSP	
	No.	%	No.	%	No.	%
Fetal outcome						
Fetal loss	7	17	19	31	9	50
Prematurity	11	27	13	21	7	39
Term	22	55	28	47	2	11
Maternal outcome	⌐────────── * ──────────⌐					
			⌐──── *** ────⌐			
Impaired renal function	9	23	10	17	11	65
Hypertension						
Total	21	52	28	47	12	70
Irreversible	6	15	5	8	4	23
Early	8	20	16	27	9	53
Severe	7	17	9	15	4	23
Increased proteinuria						
Total	29	72	33	56	12	70
Irreversible	2	5	6	10	4	23
			⌐──── ** ────⌐			
'Bad' maternal outcome	13	33	18	31	12	71

DMP, diffuse mesangial proliferation; FSHS, focal and segmental hyalinosis and sclerosis; FSP, focal and segmental proliferative (including crescents).
*$P<0.05$, **$P<0.025$, *** $P<0.01$.

Table 6.6.2–6 Fetal and maternal outcome of women with IgA nephropathy and superimposed lesions on renal biopsy (from Packham et al 1988a, with permission)

	≥10% sclerosed glomeruli (18 women)		Active crescents (8 women)		Severe vessel lesions (10 women)	
	No. of fetuses	%	No. of fetuses	%	No. of fetuses	%
Fetal outcome						
Fetal loss	12	36	4	36	13	54
Prematurity	11	33	4	36	6	25
Term	10	30	3	28	5	21
Total	33	100	11	100	24	100
	No. of pregnancies	%	No. of pregnancies	%	No. of pregnancies	%
Maternal outcome						
Impaired renal function	10	31	5	45	9	38
Hypertension						
Total	18	15	5	45	15	63
Irreversible	6	19	1	9	6	25
Severe	5	15	2	18	6	25
Early	11	34	4	18	10	42
Increased proteinuria						
Total	20	63	6	54	16	66
Irreversible	6	19	2	18	2	8

Table 6.6.2–7   Comparison of pregnancies in patients with and without severe vessel lesions (from Packham et al 1988a, with permission)

	Severe 10 women 24 pregnancies		Not severe 60 women 92 pregnancies	
	No.	%	No.	%
Fetal outcome	**			
Fetal loss	13	54	22	23
Prematurity	6	25	25	27
Term	5	21	47	50
Total fetuses	24	100	94	100
Maternal outcome Impaired renal function	9	38	21	23
Hypertension				
Total	10	42	14	15
Early	4	17	5	5
Increased proteinuria	16	66	65	61

**P<0.025.

associated with impaired renal function and a very poor pregnancy outcome are those with a circulating lupus anticoagulant or high anticardiolipin titre (Kincaid-Smith et al 1988).

REFERENCES

Abe S, Amagasaki Y, Konishi K et al 1985 The influence of antecedent renal disease on pregnancy. American Journal of Obstetrics and Gynecology 153: 508–514
Fairley C K, Packham D K 1989 Glomerular crescents and pregnancy. American Journal of Kidney Diseases 13: 250–252
Fairley K F, Whitworth J A, Kincaid-Smith P 1973 Glomerulonephritis and pregnancy. In: P Kincaid-Smith, T H Mathew, E L Becker (eds) Glomerulonephritis. Wiley, New York, pp 871–890
Jungers P, Forget D, Henry-Amar M et al 1986 Chronic kidney disease and pregnancy. In: J P Grunfeld, M H Maxwell, J F Bach et al (eds) Advances in nephrology. Year Book Medical Publishers, Chicago, vol 15: p 103–137
Kida H, Takeda S, Yokoyama H et al 1985 Focal glomerular sclerosis in preeclampsia. Clinical Nephrology 24: 221–227
Kincaid-Smith P (ed) 1975 The kidney — a clinicopathological study. Blackwell Scientific, Oxford
Kincaid-Smith P, Fairley K F 1987 Renal disease in pregnancy. Three controversial areas: mesangial IgA nephropathy, focal glomerular sclerosis (focal and segmental hyalinosis and sclerosis), and reflux nephropathy. American Journal of Kidney Diseases 9: 328–333
Kincaid-Smith P, Nicholls K 1983 Mesangial IgA nephropathy. American Journal of Kidney Diseases 3: 90–94
Kincaid-Smith P, Whitworth J A (eds) 1987 The kidney, 2nd edn. Blackwell Scientific, Oxford
Kincaid-Smith P, Mathew T H, Becker E L (eds) 1973 Proceedings International Symposium on Glomerulonephritis, Melbourne 1972. Wiley, New York
Kincaid-Smith P, Whitworth J A, Fairley K F 1980 Mesangial IgA nephropathy in pregnancy. Clinical and Experimental Hypertension 2: 821–838
Kincaid-Smith P, Kloss M, Fairley K F 1988 Lupus anticoagulant associated with renal thrombotic microangiopathy and pregnancy-related renal failure. Quarterly Journal of Medicine 258: 795–815
Nagai Y, Arai Y, Washizawa Y et al 1991 Fsas-like lesions in preeclampsia. Clinical Nephrology 36: 134–140
Nicholls K M, Fairley K F, Dowling J P et al 1984 The clinical course of mesangial IgA nephropathy. Quarterly Journal of Medicine 53: 227–250
Nicholls K M, Walker R G, Dowling J P et al 1985 'Malignant' nephropathy. American Journal of Kidney Diseases 5: 42–49
Nochy D, Nihglais N, Jacquot C et al 1986 De novo focal glomerulosclerosis in preeclampsia. Clinical Nephrology 25:1–85
Packham D, Whitworth J A, Fairley K F et al 1988a Histological features of IgA glomerulonephritis as predictors of pregnancy outcome. Clinical Nephrology 30: 22–26
Packham D, North R A, Fairley K F et al 1988b IgA glomerulonephritis and pregnancy. Clinical Nephrology 30: 15–21
Surian M, Imbasciati E, Cosci P et al 1984 Glomerular disease and pregnancy. Nephron 36: 101–105
Whitworth J A, Kincaid-Smith P, Fairley K F 1982 The outcome of pregnancy in mesangial IgA nephropathy. In: M B Sammour, E M Symonds, F P Zuspan, N El-Tomi (eds) Pregnancy hypertension. Ain Shams University Press, Egypt, ch 49, pp 403–408

6.6.3   Membranous glomerulonephritis and pregnancy

Membranous glomerulonephritis has well defined morphological features (Fig. 6.6.3–1) and has a benign course in women. In our experience, progression to renal failure is an exceptional event in women with membranous glomerulonephritis (Murphy et al 1988). Against this background and because crescent formation is extremely rare in membranous glomerulonephritis outside the context of pregnancy, this form of glomerulonephritis provides a good model for the study of the effects of pregnancy on glomerulonephritis.

We have published our experience in membranous glomerulonephritis which has been accumulated over a 30 year period (Packham et al 1987). Only one other large series of cases has been reported (Jungers et al 1986).

We studied 33 pregnancies in 24 patients with

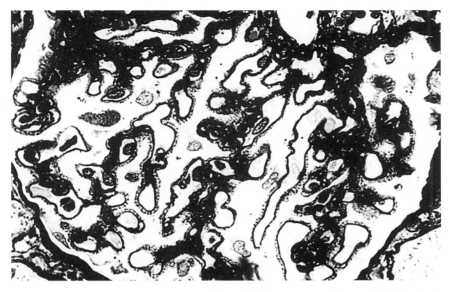

Fig. 6.6.3–1   Characteristic spike formation on the outer surface of the basement membrane, the hallmark of membranous glomerulonephritis.

membranous glomerulonephritis. Fetal loss including therapeutic abortions occurred in 24% of pregnancies and 43% of fetuses were premature.

Maternal renal function declined during pregnancy in 3 patients (9% of pregnancies), and in 2 patients renal function remained impaired after pregnancy. The clinical course in these 3 patients has been recorded previously (Kincaid-Smith 1975, 1984).

Hypertension was recorded in pregnancy in 48% of cases and in 3 women de novo hypertension did not resolve by 6 months post partum.

Proteinuria increased significantly in 55% of cases, and in 6 women (25%) this increase in proteinuria had not returned to prepregnancy levels by 6 months after pregnancy. Nephrotic range proteinuria in the first trimester was strongly associated with a poor outcome for the fetus ($P<0.0004$) and mother ($P<0.0002$) (Packham et al 1987).

Birth weights were available for 20 of 25 live births and 7 (33%) were small for gestational age (Fig. 6.6.3–2).

Remarkably small numbers of pregnancies have been recorded in women with membranous glomerulonephritis. Table 6.6.3–1 shows all the available published details on women with mem-

branous glomerulonephritis who undertook pregnancy.

In the only two large series, our own and that of Jungers et al (1986), the results were similar with a 35% of total fetal loss recorded by Jungers and a 24% total fetal loss in our series. Maternal results are also similar both in Jungers' series and in others recorded in Table 6.6.3–1.

Nephrotic syndrome developed in pregnancy in 35% of Jungers' cases and in 36% of our cases. In one of the early series, that of Studd & Blainey (1969), all patients were nephrotic in all pregnancies. Nephrotic syndrome was a strong determinant of a poor maternal and fetal outcome in our series (Table 6.6.3–2). Studd & Blainey (1969) recorded hypertension in 83% of pregnancies, whereas 45% of our patients were hypertensive.

The interpretation of the influence of pregnancy on the natural history of the membranous glomerulonephritis differs between the different authors who have contributed in this field.

Because our published experience in membranous glomerulonephritis in women (Murphy et al 1988) is of a benign disorder which almost never progresses to renal failure, we were concerned that 2 of 3 women with membranous

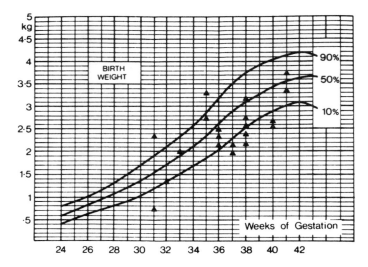

Fig. 6.6.3–2   Birth weights of infants of 20 patients with membranous glomerulonephritis.

glomerulonephritis whose renal function deteriorated during the 9 month period of gestation had not recovered the function which they had lost by 6 months post partum. This is clearly quite different from our experience of the natural history of membranous glomerulonephritis and we would attribute the deterioration, which occurred during pregnancy and persisted, to the effects of pregnancy. We were particularly persuaded that pregnancy had caused the deterioration because we demonstrated the development of superimposed crescents in 1 of the 2 patients who deteriorated — a complication which we have never observed in women with membranous glomerulonephritis except during pregnancy. In the other patient we demonstrated superimposed segmental hyalinosis and sclerosis accompanying marked deterioration in renal function during pregnancy.

These 2 patients are documented in detail because of the importance of the question. Does pregnancy influence the natural history of glomerulonephritis?

In the first, whose course is illustrated in Fig.

Table 6.6.3–1   Summary of published data on membranous glomerulonephritis and pregnancy

	Studd & Blainey 1969	Forland & Spargo 1969	Noel et al 1979	Katz et al 1980	Klockars et al 1980	Surian et al 1984	Abe et al 1985	Jungers et al 1986	Packham et al 1987
No. of patients	6	4	7	7	6	7	7	18	24
No. of pregnancies	12	6	9	10	9	8	13	37	33
Therapeutic abortions	2	1	1	–	0	–	0	3	4
Spontaneous abortions	0	2	0	0	1	0	0	8	3
Stillbirths	0	0	1	0	0	0	1	2	1
Neonatal deaths	0	0	0	0	0	0	0	0	0
Total fetal loss	2	3	2	0	1	0	1	13	8
% fetal loss	16	50	22	0	11	0	8	35	24
Renal function irreversible	0	0	0	0	0	0	–	0	2
Renal function reversible	0	0	0	0	0	1	–	1	1
Hypertension (diastolic pressure ≥90 mmHg)	10	0	0	5	1	0	–	13	15
Nephrotic in pregnancy	12	3	–	5	2	–		13	12

Table 6.6.3–2 Correlation between nephrotic range proteinuria in first trimester and fetal and maternal outcome using Fisher's exact test (from Packham et al 1987, with permission)

Fetal outcome	Poor	Good
Proteinuria >5 g/24 h in first trimester	8	2
Proteinuria <5 g/24 h in first trimester	2	21

Poor fetal outcome = fetal loss or <32 weeks' gestation. Good fetal outcome = live infant born after 32 weeks' gestation. *P*<0.0004.

Maternal outcome	Poor	Good
Proteinuria >5 g/24 h in first trimester	10	0
Proteinuria <5 g/24 h in first trimester	7	16

Good maternal outcome = no development of renal impairment or irreversible hypertension or proteinuria in pregnancy. Poor maternal outcome = development of renal impairment or of irreversible hypertension or proteinuria in pregnancy. *P*<0.0002.

when the blood pressure was normal, showed a very mild membranous lesion, so mild that the membranous change was missed on the initial histological evaluation. Serum creatinine was normal at that time but deteriorated strikingly across the period of gestation as the blood pressure rose from normal levels to a level of 190/130 and became refractory to treatment. Urine protein rose from a trace to 15 g/24 h during the course of pregnancy. A biopsy at the end of pregnancy showed crescents in many glomeruli. Although the membranous lesion and the crescents resolved with treatment, renal function remained impaired for 2 further years. Without aggressive treatment of both her hypertension and crescentic glomerular disease this patient might have been expected to progress to end stage renal failure, which we would have attributed to the effects of the pregnancy on the course of the membranous glomerulonephritis because:

6.6.3–3, we have no doubt that pregnancy had an adverse effect on the course of membranous glomerulonephritis. A renal biopsy at 4 months,

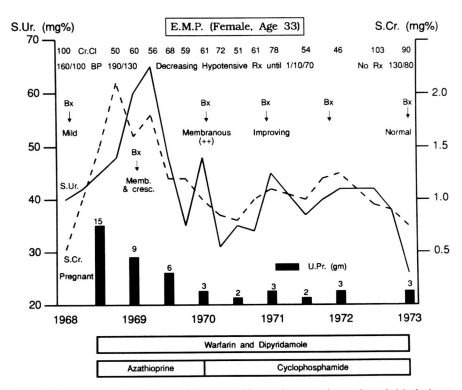

Fig. 6.6.3–3   Course during pregnancy in a 33 year old woman with membranous glomerulonephritis during pregnancy and in the subsequent 5 years.

1. Histology was shown to deteriorate dramatically during pregnancy with the considerable increase in the membranous lesions and development of crescents and subsequent sclerosis of glomeruli
2. Severe hypertension, an unusual event in women with membranous glomerulonephritis, developed during pregnancy
3. Proteinuria appeared for the first time during pregnancy and progressed to a frank nephrotic syndrome
4. Renal function deteriorated during pregnancy

Crescent formation, as noted above, is an exceptional event in the course of membranous glomerulonephritis. As indicated in Figure 6.6.3–3, we have a policy of frequent renal biopsies to document the reason for clinical changes and, in numerous repeat biopsies in 139 patients with membranous glomerulonephritis, only 4 patients developed crescents; 3 of these were women who developed superimposed crescents during pregnancy at a time when they had other evidence of deterioration in renal function. One man developed crescents when an episode of clearly documented postinfectious glomerulonephritis was superimposed on a preexisting membranous lesion.

The second patient with membranous glomerulonephritis, who suffered irreversible deterioration in renal function, had had stable renal function for 8 years prior to her pregnancy. Renal function deteriorated abruptly during pregnancy in association with extensive superimposed lesion of focal and segmental hyalinosis and sclerosis. Serum creatinine doubled during pregnancy. It had not fallen by 6 months after pregnancy but stabilized at 0.4 mmol/l on treatment with azathioprine, warfarin and dipyridamole. Renal function abruptly deteriorated and progressed to end stage renal failure when the above treatment was withdrawn 4 years later. In this patient we would regard this sequence of events as evidence that pregnancy had an adverse effect on the course of membranous glomerulonephritis.

While we would regard these 2 patients as examples of a clear cut and deleterious effect of pregnancy on the course of membranous glome-

rulonephritis, other workers with seemingly worse results in individual patients have not judged them to reflect the effect of the pregnancy on the course of the membranous glomerulonephritis.

Studd (1977) states that his previous series (Studd & Blainey 1969) showed that the prognosis in chronic renal disease is excellent in the absence of hypertension. When we consider his 1969 report, however, the largest subgroup of 6 patients had membranous glomerulonephritis. All were hypertensive in pregnancy, blood pressures being recorded in late pregnancy as 150/100, 190/120, 200/120, 160/100, 250/150, and 160/100 in the 6 patients. Where the blood pressure was recorded in early pregnancy in these patients, it was normal or very much lower than the level in late pregnancy. Our conclusion would therefore be that the pregnancy caused the severe hypertension and if that were true then the mere level of blood pressure recorded surely represents a deleterious effect of pregnancy. In view of the height of the blood pressure, it is no surprise to read that 2 of the 6 patients subsequently died of malignant hypertension and because this commenced in pregnancy and is a rare event in membranous glomerulonephritis we would attribute these deaths to the pregnancies.

The membranous form of lupus glomerulonephritis is histologically so similar to idiopathic membranous glomerulonephritis that a comparison of the results in these two forms of glomerulonephritis in pregnancy is warranted.

Tables 6.6.3–3 and 6.6.3–4 show the fetal and maternal outcome in 33 pregnancies in idiopathic membranous glomerulonephritis and 16 pregnancies in lupus membranous glomerulonephritis. The results are surprisingly similar as far as fetal outcome is concerned.

In many respects the maternal outcome seems to be more serious in idiopathic glomerulonephritis than in lupus membranous glomerulonephritis. There was more irreversible impairment of renal function in the idiopathic group and hypertension was present in 46% of pregnancies in idiopathic membranous glomerulonephritis compared with 25% of pregnancies in patients with membranous lupus glomerulonephritis. An increase in proteinuria was also more frequent in the idiopathic groups (Table 6.6.3–4).

Table 6.6.3–3   Comparison of fetal outcome between patients with idiopathic membranous and lupus membranous glomerulonephritis (from Packham et al 1992 with permission)

	Idiopathic membranous glomerulonephritis (*n* = 33)		Lupus membranous glomerulonephritis (*n* = 16)	
	No.	%	No.	%
Therapeutic abortion	4	12	1	6
Spontaneous abortion	3	9	3	19
Stillbirth	1	3		
Neonatal death	–			
Total fetal loss	8	24	4	25
Severe prematurity	2	6	1	6
Prematurity	12	36	4	25
Term	11	33	7	44

Table 6.6.3–4   Comparison of maternal outcome between patients with idiopathic membranous and lupus membranous glomerulonephritis (from Packham et al 1992 with permission)

	Idiopathic membranous glomerulonephritis (*n* = 33)		Lupus membranous glomerulonephritis (*n* = 16)	
	No.	%	No.	%
Irreversible renal impairment	2	6	0	
Reversible renal impairment	1	3	1	6
Total renal impairment	3	9	1	6
Hypertension irreversible	3	9	2	13
Hypertension reversible	12	36	2	13
Total hypertension	15	46	4	25
Increased proteinuria irreversible	6	18	3	19
Increased proteinuria reversible	12	36	3	19
Total increased proteinuria	18	55	6	38
Nephrotic	12	26	4	25

An interesting feature of membranous glomerulonephritis is that like other immunologically mediated disorders such as systemic lupus erythematosus, Graves' disease and myasthenia gravis, membranous glomerulonephritis can be induced in the fetal kidney presumably by transplacental transfer of maternal antibodies (Nauta et al 1990).

REFERENCES

Abe S, Amagaski Y, Konishi K et al 1985 The influence of antecedent renal disease on pregnancy. American Journal of Obstetrics and Gynecology 153: 508–514

Forland M, Spargo B 1969 Clinicopathological correlations in idiopathic nephrotic syndrome with membranous nephropathy. Nephron 6: 498

Jungers P, Forget D, Henry-Amar M et al 1986 Chronic kidney disease and pregnancy. In: J P Grunfeld, M H Maxwell, J F Bach et al (eds) Advances in nephrology. Year Book Medical Publishers, Chicago, vol 15: 103–141

Katz A I, Davison J M, Hayslett J P et al 1980 Pregnancy in women with kidney disease. Kidney International 18: 192–206

Kincaid-Smith P 1984 The kidney in pregnancy (Proceedings, Second Asian Pacific Congress of Nephrology 1983). The Dominion Press–Hedges and Bell, Maryborough, p 228

Kincaid-Smith P (ed) 1975 The kidney: a clinicopathologic study. Blackwell Scientific, Oxford p 222

Klockers M, Saarikoski S, Ikonen E et al 1980 Pregnancy in patients with renal disease. Acta Medica Scandinavica 207: 207

Murphy B F, Fairley K F, Kincaid-Smith P 1988 Idiopathic membranous glomerulonephritis: long-term follow-up 139 cases. Clinical Nephrology 30: 175–181

Nagai Y, Arai Y, Washizawa Y et al 1991 FSGS-like lesions in preeclampsia. Clinical Nephrology 36: 134–140

Nauta J, de Heer E, Baldwin W M et al 1990 Transplacental induction of membranous nephropathy in a neonate. Pediatric Nephrology 4: 111–116

Noel L H, Zanetti M, Droz D et al 1979 Long-term prognosis of idiopathic membranous glomerulonephritis. Study on 116 untreated patients. American Journal of Medicine 66:82

Packham D K, North R A, Fairley K F et al 1987 Membranous glomerulonephritis and pregnancy. Clinical Nephrology 28: 56–64

Packham D K, Lam S S, Nicholls K et al 1992 Lupus nephritis and pregnancy. Quarterly Journal of Medicine 83: 315–324

Rovati C, Perrino M L, Barbiano Di Belgiojoso G et al 1984 Pregnancy and course of primary glomerulonephritis. Contributions to Nephrology 37: 182–189

Studd J W W 1977 Chronic renal disease in pregnancy. Panminerva Medica 19: 389–390

Studd J W W, Blainey J D 1969 Pregnancy and the nephrotic syndrome. British Medical Journal 1: 276–280

Surian M, Imbasciati E, Cosci P et al 1984 Glomerular disease and pregnancy. Study of 123 pregnancies in patients with primary and secondary glomerular diseases. Nephron 36: 101–105

6.6.4 Focal and segmental hyalinosis and sclerosis

There are difficulties in analysing the results of pregnancy in this form of glomerulonephritis the light microscopic appearance of which is shown in Figure 6.6.4–1.

A major difficulty concerns the very close simi-larity between the lesions of severe preeclampsia and those of focal and segmental hyalinosis. (Kincaid-Smith & Fairley 1987). Figure 4.5.2–11 shows florid glomerular lesion seen in a patient with preeclampsia. This lesion may be virtually indistinguishable from the lesion of segmental hyalinosis described by Habib et al (1961, 1970) as 'hyalinose focal et segmentaire' in children with the nephrotic syndrome. More recently the interpretation which has been placed on this histological resemblance is that lesions of focal and segmental hyalinosis occur as a complication of preeclampsia (Kida et al 1985, Nochy et al 1986). The recent publication by Nagai et al (1991) is useful in that it suggests, as we have always believed, that the segmental hyalinosis/sclerosis lesions occur in association with severe pre-eclampsia. These authors found a strong correla-tion between hyalinosis/sclerosis lesions and the presence of granulated glomerular epithelial cells which we have also shown correlate with the severity of preeclampsia (Kincaid-Smith et al 1985). In addition they found a strong correlation between segmental hyalinosis/sclerosis and double contours in glomerular capillaries, another lesion which we first identified as a manifestation of severe preeclampsia (Kincaid-Smith 1973, 1975). Segmental hyalinosis/sclerosis also correlated strongly with the degree of proteinuria and with its

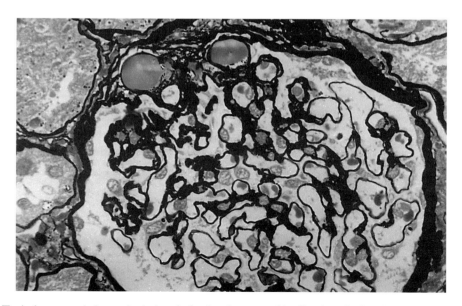

Fig. 6.6.4–1 Typical segmental glomerular lesions in focal and segmental hyalinosis and sclerosis.

duration after delivery. These clinical manifestations also reflect severe preeclampsia.

The lesion illustrated in Figure 4.5.2–11 is essentially a large hyaline subendothelial deposit. Similar deposits in adjacent capillaries in the same glomerulus less closely resemble segmental hyalinosis because they do not fill the whole capillary (Fig. 4.5.2–7) or because they are fibrinoid containing fibrillar fibrin which can be identified on its ultrastructural characteristics (Fig. 4.5.2–2).

The similarity of these lesions illustrates the dilemma of the pathologist in distinguishing the lesions of severe preeclampsia from those of focal and segmental hyalinosis. The only features in Figure 4.5.2–11 which differ from segmental hyalinosis seen in the nephrotic syndrome is that there is no adhesion to Bowman's capsule and that epithelial cells are less damaged, showing some distinct foot processes.

We described superimposed lesions of focal and segmental hyalinosis developing during pregnancy and disappearing after pregnancy in a patient with healed membranous glomerulonephritis many years ago (Kincaid-Smith 1975). This development of segmental hyalinosis is best demonstrated in mesangial IgA glomerulonephritis as illustrated in Table 6.6.2–4.

Because the lesions of severe preeclampsia can so closely resemble those of focal and segmental hyalinosis this creates difficulties in classification of biopsies done during pregnancy or in the early postpartum period as to whether the changes illustrated in Figure 4.5.2–11 indicate an underlying glomerulonephritis of the focal and segmental hyalinosis and sclerosis category or whether they represent the changes of preeclampsia.

Because of these difficulties we have included in this analysis of the outcome of pregnancy in primary focal and segmental hyalinosis and sclerosis only those patients whose biopsy, on which the diagnosis was based, was performed prior to 16 weeks' gestation or at a time remote from the pregnancy. We also required persistent proteinuria for a year after pregnancy as a criterion for inclusion.

Applying the above criteria, we were able to identify a group of 21 patients who undertook 31 pregnancies between 1961 and 1987 under our care.

The methods used and definitions were as outlined in 6.6.

Because this is a small group of patients and because the outcome of pregnancy is particularly poor in this group, the full details of individual patients are given in Table 6.6.4–1. Fetal outcome is shown in Table 6.6.4–2.

Fetal loss was very high, occurring in 14 pregnancies (45%); 11 (35%) of these occurred in late pregnancy, and included 5 stillbirths and 6 neonatal deaths as a complication of severe superimposed preeclampsia. There were 2 spontaneous abortions and 1 therapeutic abortion.

Prematurity (71%) and severe prematurity (23%) were common among surviving infants

The birth weights showed that 29% of babies were small for gestational age (Packham et al 1988).

In this group of patients, where results were particularly poor, the question of the influence of presentation during pregnancy with a pregnancy related complication was examined.

Table 6.6.4–3 separates the pregnancies into those where the diagnosis was known prior to pregnancy, of which there were only 10, and those made during or after the pregnancy (21). This latter group included a high proportion of patients who presented during pregnancy with complications of pregnancy. Although overall fetal loss is similar, perinatal mortality was higher in patients in whom the diagnosis was made during or after pregnancy (48% compared with 10% in those with a diagnosis prior to pregnancy).

The maternal outcome in these patients was also worse than that in other histological categories of glomerulonephritis. It was partly our experience in individual patients in this group that caused us to view the outcome of glomerulonephritis in pregnancy as unpredictable and potentially very serious (Kincaid-Smith et al 1967). Consider the case of CH (Table 6.6.4–1). This young woman, with a history of a nephritic illness as a child, presented to us in early pregnancy with normal renal function, a normal blood pressure, a trace of protein in the urine and a benign urine deposit. By 25 weeks' gestation she had developed severe hypertension, and the nephrotic syndrome and renal function had declined. A biopsy at this stage showed extensive acute lesions of focal and segmental hyalinosis together with severe vessel lesions.

Table 6.6.4–1 Summary of clinical course and pregnancies of 21 women with primary focal and segmental hyalinosis and sclerosis (from Packham et al 1988, with permission)

Patient	Year of pregnancy	Treatment in pregnancy	Pregnancy outcome	Initial renal biopsy	Clinical course post partum
TT	86	Heparin, steroids, plasma exchange	Neonatal death: induced 28 weeks. Irreversible deterioration in renal function. Irreversible, early hypertension. Irreversible increase in proteinuria. Nephrotic	8 weeks' pregnant: 1/16 sclerosed, 10/16 FSHS, mild vessel lesions	Chronic renal failure/persistent nephrotic range proteinuria 1 year post partum. Creatinine 0.37 mmol/l
DC	86		Stillbirth: 26 weeks, 580g. Reversible impairment renal function. Severe, early, reversible hypertension. Reversible increased proteinuria. Nephrotic	2 weeks post partum: 2/12 sclerosed, mild vessel lesions	Persistent proteinuria 1 year post partum
KV	86		Live birth: 34 weeks. Severe, early, reversible hypertension. Eclampsia Reversible, increased proteinuria	8 months post partum: 2/30 sclerosed, 5 FSHS, mild vessel lesions	Persistent proteinuria
SG	85		Neonatal death: induced 26 weeks, 460 g. Reversible impairment renal function. Severe, early, reversible hypertension. Reversible increase in proteinuria	12 months post partum: 0/44 sclerosed, 2/44 FSHS, moderate vessel lesions	Persistent proteinuria 1 year post partum
HW	85		Stillbirth: 26 weeks, 710 g. Reversible impairment renal function. Severe, early, reversible hypertension. Reversible increase in proteinuria. Nephrotic	12 months post partum: 0/20 sclerosed 1/20 FSHS	Proteinuria resolved after 6 months post partum
CG	85		Stillbirth: 31 weeks, 1025 g. Severe, early, reversible hypertension. Reversible increased proteinuria. Nephrotic	6 months post partum: 1/30 sclerosed, 6 FSHS, mild vessel lesions	Persistent glomerular haematuria
MB 1	84		Live birth: induced 32 weeks, 1540 g. Reversible impairment renal function and hypertension. Stable proteinuria	16 weeks' pregnant (2), 12 months post partum (1): 2/60 sclerosed, 1/60 FSHS mild vessel lesions	Stable proteinuria persists 2 years post partum
2	85	Heparin	Live birth: 35 weeks, 2119 g. Reversible impairment renal function. Normotensive. Stable proteinuria		
EJ	84		Live birth: 37 weeks. Reversible increase in proteinuria	5 months post partum: 7/15 sclerosed, 3 FSHS, mild renal lesions	Persistent proteinuria

Table 6.6.4–1 (*contd*)

Patient		Year of pregnancy	Treatment in pregnancy	Pregnancy outcome	Initial renal biopsy	Clinical course post partum
SB	1	84		Live birth: 27 weeks, 1141 g. Severe, early, reversible hypertension. Reversible increased proteinuria	7 months post partum: 1/38 sclerosed, mild vessel lesions	Persistent glomerular haematuria only
	2	85		Live birth: 35 weeks' gestation, 3060 g. No problems		
	3	86		Therapeutic abortion at 10 weeks. Social/psychiatric indications		
VL		83		Stillbirth: 27 weeks, 600 g Reversible impairment renal function. Severe, early, reversible increased proteinuria. Nephrotic	6 months post 1/10 sclerosed, 3/10 FSHS mild vessel lesions	Had been diagnosed 10 years prior to pregnancy. Persistent proteinuria post partum
VG		83		Livebirth: 31 weeks. Reversible impairment renal function. Severe, early, reversible hypertension. Reversible increased proteinuria	6 months post partum: repeated 3 years post partum: 2/25 sclerosed, mild vessel lesions	Persistent proteinuria
EO	1	81		Live birth: 38 weeks. Severe, early, reversible hypertension. Reversible increase in proteinuria.	11 months post partum: 2/20 sclerosed, 4/20 lesions of FSHS, mild renal lesions	Persistent proteinuria 6 years post partum
	2	85	Heparin	Live birth: 34 weeks. Reversible hypertension. Reversible increase in proteinuria		
SC	1	80		Neonatal death: induced 27 weeks. Severe, early, reversible hypertension. Reversible increase in proteinuria. Nephrotic	14 months post partum: 3/20 FSHS lesion, mild vessel lesions	Proteinuria resolved 1 year post partum but repeat biopsy at 16 weeks' gestation in 85 pregnancy 2/28 FSHS
	2	85	Heparin	Live birth: 37 weeks, 2400 g. Reversible hypertension and proteinuria		
AE		80		Live birth: 38 weeks. Exacerbation of hypertension	18 months post partum: 14/30 sclerosed, 2 FSHS, mild vessel lesions	Hypertension persistent
MK	1	78		Live birth: 33 weeks, 2538 g. Severe, early, reversible hypertension. Reversible increased proteinuria. Nephrotic	10 weeks' pregnant: 1/30 sclerosed, 4 FSHS, mild vessel lesions	Persistent glomerular haematuria
	2	80		Neonatal death: 26 weeks, 850 g. Reversible impairment of renal function. Severe, early, reversible hypertension. Reversible		

Table 6.6.4–1 (contd)

Patient		Year of pregnancy	Treatment in pregnancy	Pregnancy outcome	Initial renal biopsy	Clinical course post partum
				increased proteinuria. Nephrotic		
JG	1	78		Live birth: 37 weeks, 2910 g Glomerular haematuria only	17 weeks' pregnant: 6/17 sclerosed areas FSHS, mild vessel lesions	Persistent glomerular haematuria
JS	1	77		Neonatal death: 28 weeks, 1100 g. Reversible impairment renal function. Severe, early, irreversible hypertension. Reversible increase in proteinuria	4 months post partum 78: 0/10 sclerosed, 1 FSHS. Repeat 24 months post partum: 1/40 sclerosed, 7/40 FSHS, mild vessel lesions	Persistent hypertension and proteinuria at 10 years follow up
	2	80		Live birth: 37 weeks, 3275 g. Stable hypertension on Aldomet.		
	3	85		Spontaneous abortions at 10 weeks' gestation		
	4	86				
	5	87	Dipy-ridamole	Live birth: induced 28 weeks, 706 g Reversible impairment of renal function. Early exacerbation of hypertension. Reversible increase in proteinuria		
GD		77		Stillbirth: 30 weeks' gestation. Early irreversible hypertension. Reversible increased proteinuria	6 months post partum: 1/10 sclerosed	Persistent hypertension and proteinuria
CH		64		Neonatal death: 25 weeks' gestation. Irreversible renal impairment. Severe, early, reversible hypertension. Irreversible increased proteinuria. Nephrotic	25 weeks' pregnant: focal hyalinosis and sclerosis. Advanced vessel lesions	ESRF 2 years post partum
BW		62		Live birth: 34 weeks' gestation. Irreversible renal impairment. Severe, early, irreversible hypertension. Irreversible increased proteinuria. Nephrotic	1 month post partum: focal hyalinosis lesions. Repeat 3 years post partum: similar	ESRF7 years post partum
RE		62		Live birth: 36 weeks' gestation. Irreversible renal impairment. Early, reversible hypertension. Reversible increased proteinuria.	14 weeks' pregnant: focal glomerulonephritis areas of focal hyaline	ESRF 18 years later

FSHS, focal and segmental hyalinosis and sclerosis; ESRF, end stage renal failure.

Table 6.6.4–2 Fetal outcome of 31 fetuses born to 21 mothers with primary focal and segmental hyalinosis and sclerosis (from Packham et al 1988, with permission)

Fetal outcome	No. of fetuses	%
Fetal loss		
Spontaneous abortions	2	7
Therapeutic abortions	1	3
Stillbirths	5	16
Neonatal deaths	6	19
Total	14	45
Prematurity		
≤ 32 weeks' gestation	4	13
>32, >37 weeks' gestation	8	26
Total	12	39
Term	5	16
Total	31	100

In spite of immediate delivery, renal function continued to decline in the postpartum period so that she had essentially end stage renal failure shortly after pregnancy. Due to a shortage of dialysis facilities in 1964 she was maintained by rigorous conservative management on a Giordano–Giovannetti diet for 2 years prior to commencing dialysis. Two other early patients with similar lesions and normal function in early pregnancy developed the nephrotic syndrome and irreversible impairment of renal function (Kincaid-Smith et al 1967).

TT (Table 6.6.4–1), is a further patient studied and documented in detail by us, in whom we have little doubt that pregnancy had an adverse effect on the course of her renal disease. This young woman had no proteinuria 3 months prior to pregnancy. She presented at 8 weeks of gestation with the nephrotic syndrome and sclerosis of 1 glomerulus in 16 but lesions of segmental hyalinosis and sclerosis in 10 of 16 glomeruli although renal function was normal. There was no clinical response to steroids and heparin and by 26 weeks renal function had declined significantly and a biopsy showed progression of the glomerular lesions. Acute antepartum haemorrhage required induction at 27 weeks and the infant died 2 days later. Deterioration of renal function continued in the postpartum period and she required dialysis 18 months later. Clearly major deterioration occurred during pregnancy in this patient.

When we analyse our overall maternal results in patients with focal and segmental hyalinosis and sclerosis they confirm our early view that patients with this histological form of glomerulonephritis have a worse outcome than those with other forms of glomerulonephritis. The results are detailed in Table 6.6.4–4.

Of these patients 13% suffered an irreversible decline in renal function during pregnancy and almost half showed a decline in renal function during pregnancy (44%).

Table 6.6.4–3 Comparison of fetal outcome of pregnancies pre and postdating biopsy diagnosis (from Packham et al 1988, with permission)

Fetal outcome	Pre diagnosis		Post diagnosis	
	No. of foetuses	%	No. of foetuses	%
Fetal loss				
Spontaneous abortions	0	–	1	10
Therapeutic abortions	0	–	2	20
Stillbirths	5	24	0	–
Neonatal deaths	5	24	1	10
Total	10	48	4	40
Prematurity				
≤32 weeks' gestation	3	14	1	10
>32, <37 weeks' gestation	5	24	3	30
Total	8	38	4	20
Term	3	14	2	20
Total	21	100	10	100

Table 6.6.4–4 Maternal outcome of 32 pregnancies undertaken by 21 women with primary focal and segmental hyalinosis and sclerosis (from Packham et al 1988, with permission)

Maternal outcome	No. of pregnancies	%
Impaired renal function		
Irreversible	4	13
Reversible	11	36
Total	15	49
Hypertension		
Irreversible	4	13
Reversible	17	55
Exacerbation	2	6
Total hypertensive pregnancies	23	74
Stable	3	10
Severe	14	61
Proteinuria		
Irreversible	3	10
Reversible	19	61
Total increased proteinuria	22	71
Stable proteinuria	5	16
Nephrotic range proteinuria	13	42

Hypertension developed de novo in pregnancy in 68% of cases and was irreversible in 13% and severe in 45%.

Proteinuria increased in 71% of pregnancies and was irreversible in 10%. Nephrotic range proteinuria was documented in 42% of cases.

One of the difficulties in comparing our results with those of other groups concerns the histological lesion. Other groups use the nomenclature focal glomerulosclerosis. What the term focal glomerular sclerosis means is global sclerosis (not hyalinosis) of some glomeruli and not others (Churg & Sobin 1982). Such lesions are non-specific and occur in a wide variety of renal lesions. The essential lesions in focal and segmental hyalinosis are segmental, involving segments of the glomerular tuft rather than the whole glomerular tuft (Fig. 6.6.4–1). Although global sclerosis does occur, it is non-specific.

In our view it is the segmental hyalinosis which is the early and characteristic lesion in this form of glomerulonephritis. Contrast the appearance in Figure 4.5.2–11, which shows hyalinosis, with the electron microscopic picture of sclerosis

(Fig. 6.6.4–2), which typically shows collapse and thickening of the basement membrane capillary and collapse of capillaries with disappearance of the lumen. Although sclerosis is seen in focal and segmental hyalinosis and sclerosis, it is more frequently encountered as a scar following healing of a segmental proliferative lesion or crescent. Few authors discussing the results of pregnancy in what they call focal sclerosis or focal glomerulosclerosis describe in detail which specific lesions they used to place patients in this histological category. This leads to considerable confusion as to which form of glomerulonephritis is being studied.

In a small series of 10 pregnancies in 6 patients with 'primary focal glomerulosclerosis', Jungers et al (1987) recorded a high rate of fetal complications but no deterioration in renal function in the mothers. Barcelo et al (1986) reported 17 pregnancies in 13 women with 'focal glomerulosclerosis' and recorded prematurity in 3 pregnancies and an abortion in 1. Surian documented 25 pregnancies in 19 women with 'focal glomerulosclerosis' and reported late fetal loss

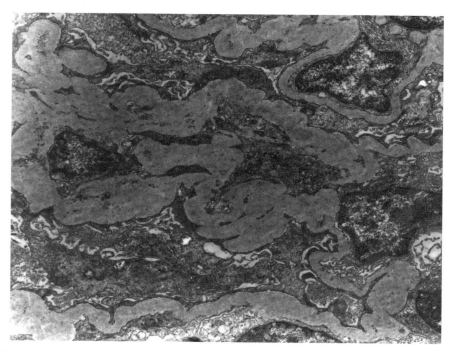

Fig. 6.6.4–2   Electron microscopic appearance of sclerosis — glomerular capillaries are collapsed and basement membranes are thickened.

(2 fetal deaths in utero and 4 perinatal deaths) in 24%. Hypertension in pregnancy was frequent but they recorded no rapid deterioration in renal function (Surian et al 1984).

Perhaps the most likely reason why our own experience appears to be worse from that recorded by Barcelo et al (1986), Surian et al (1984) and Jungers et al (1987) is that the majority of the pregnancies which we studied were in women who presented during pregnancy with a pregnancy related complication, whereas the other authors analysed the overall outcome in pregnancy in women attending their renal clinics in whom the diagnosis of 'focal glomerulosclerosis' was presumably made prior to pregnancy. In 6.6.8 we discuss the influence of presentation during pregnancy on outcome in patients with glomerulonephritis. Clearly in a unit such as ours, which has been a tertiary referral centre for complicated pregnancies for 30 years, the patient population is different from that attending a nephrology service.

Gaber & Spargo (1987) discuss the lesion of focal and segmental glomerulosclerosis in some detail. They searched for lesions of focal/segmental glomerulosclerosis in 20 biopsies performed between 1979 and 1983 on atypical or severe cases of preeclampsia. Lesions of pregnancy induced hypertension or preeclampsia were present in 19 of 20 biopsies. Lesions of focal segmental glomerular sclerosis were present in 7 cases in 2–10% of glomeruli.

Vascular lesions were documented in the biopsies and in 5 of these the biopsy also showed focal segmental glomerulosclerosis. Tubular interstitial changes were observed in 10 cases, 6 of which also showed focal segmental glomerulosclerosis.

Their conclusion from this study was that lesions of focal segmental glomerulosclerosis were ischaemic in nature. They cautioned against confusing the form of focal segmental glomerulosclerosis which they documented in biopsies of women with severe preeclampsia with the primary form of focal segmental glomerulosclerosis, and quote Cameron's series as describing a progressive unremittent course in primary cases with a 10 year survival of 38% (Cameron et al 1978). The interstitial and vascular lesions illustrated by Gaber & Spargo (1987) are very similar to those

which we have described in reflux nephropathy (Kincaid-Smith 1984), and in most of our patients with similar lesions to those which they describe and illustrate we would be able to document overt or occult evidence of reflux nephropathy using imaging techniques (Kincaid-Smith 1991). We have specifically excluded patients with reflux nephropathy or other secondary forms of focal and segmental hyalinosis and sclerosis from our own analysis of results during pregnancy in which we include only primary glomerular lesions.

In terms of what is said to be 'the usual unremitting progressive course of the primary form of focal and segmental glomerular sclerosis' (Cameron et al 1978), we have recorded our experience in adults with primary focal and segmental hyalinosis. In this group of adults our results differed from Cameron's (Cameron et al 1978). Many of Cameron's patients were children in whom the course seems to be a more progressive one. In our adult women 93% survived for 10 years (Kincaid-Smith & Yeung 1979). This contrasts with our pregnancy experience in which 3 of 5 patients followed for 10 years progressed to end stage renal failure as did TT in only 3 years. These pregnancy related complications of focal and segmental hyalinosis are not in keeping with the relatively benign natural history which we have documented in our other women with this lesion (Kincaid-Smith & Yeung 1979).

REFERENCES

Barcelo P, Lopez-Lillo J, Cabero L et al 1986 Successful pregnancy in primary glomerular disease. Kidney International 30: 914–919

Cameron J S, Turner D R, Ogg C S et al 1978 The long term prognosis of patients with focal segmental glomerulosclerosis. Clinical Nephrology 10: 213–218

Churg J, Sobin D H 1982 Renal disease. Classification and atlas of glomerular diseases. Igaku-Shoin, Tokyo, p 127–149

Gaber L W, Spargo B H 1987 Pregnancy-induced nephropathy: the significance of focal segmental glomerulosclerosis. American Journal of Kidney Diseases 9: 317–323

Habib R 1970 Classification anatomique des nephropathies glomerularies. Paediatrische Fortbildungskurse fuer die Praxis 28: 3–47

Habib R, Michielsen P, De Montera H et al 1961 Clinical microscopic and electron microscopic data in the nephrotic syndrome of unknown origin. In: Wolstenholme G E W, Cameron M P (eds) Ciba Foundation Symposium on Renal Biopsy. J & A Churchill, London

Jungers P. Forget D, Houillier P et al 1987 Pregnancy in IgA
    nephropathy, reflux nephropathy, and focal glomerular
    sclerosis. American Journal of Kidney Diseases 9: 334–338
Kida H, Takeda S, Yokoyama H et al 1985 Focal glomerular
    sclerosis in preeclampsia. Clinical Nephrology 24: 221–227
Kincaid-Smith P 1973 The similarity of lesions and
    underlying mechanism in preeclamptic toxaemia and
    postpartum renal failure. In: P Kincaid-Smith,
    T H Mathew, E L Becker (eds) Glomerulonephritis. Wiley,
    New York, p 1013–1025
Kincaid-Smith P (ed) 1975 The kidney — a
    clinicopathological study. Blackwell Scientific, Oxford, p 16
Kincaid-Smith P 1984 Diffuse parenchymal lesions in reflux
    nephropathy and the possibility of making a renal biopsy
    diagnosis in reflux nephropathy. In: C J Hodson,
    R H Heptinstall, J Winberg (eds) Reflux nephropathy
    update 1983. Contributions to nephrology. Karger, Basel,
    Vol 39: p 111–115
Kincaid-Smith P 1991 Reflux nephropathy without overt
    radiographic lesions. In: R R Bailey (ed) Proceedings of the
    Second C J Hodson Symposium on Reflux nephropathy.
    Sandoz, Christchurch
Kincaid-Smith P, Fairley K F 1987 Renal disease in
    pregnancy. Three controversial areas: mesangial IgA
    nephropathy, focal glomerular sclerosis (focal and
    segmental hyalinosis and sclerosis), and reflux
    nephropathy. American Journal of Kidney Diseases
    9: 328–333
Kincaid-Smith P, Yeung C K 1979 Focal and segmental
    proliferative glomerulonephritis, focal and segmental
    hyalinosis and sclerosis and focal sclerosis in the adult. In:
    P Kincaid-Smith, A J F d'Apice, R C Atkins (eds) Progress
    in glomerulonephritis. Wiley, New York, cha 12,
    p 231–243
Kincaid-Smith P, Fairley K F, Bullen M 1967 Kidney disease
    and pregnancy. Medical Journal of Australia 2: 1155–1159
Kincaid-Smith P, North R A, Becker G J et al 1985
    Proteinuria during pregnancy. In: V E Andreucci (ed) The
    kidney in pregnancy. Martinus Nijhoff, Boston,
    p 133–164
Nagai Y, Arai Y, Washizawa Y et al 1991 FSGS-like lesions
    in preeclampsia. Clinical Nephrology 36: 134–140
Nochy D, Hinglais N, Jacquot C et al 1986 De novo focal
    glomerular sclerosis in preeclampsia. Clinical Nephrology
    25: 116–121
Packham D K, North R A, Fairley K F et al p 1988
    Pregnancy in women with primary focal and segmental
    hyalinosis and sclerosis. Clinical Nephrology 29: 185–192
Surian M, Imbasciati E, Cosci P et al C 1984 Glomerular
    disease and pregnancy. Nephron 36: 101–105

6.6.5 Membranoproliferative glomerulonephritis (mesangiocapillary glomerulonephritis type I)

Controversy in the classification of this form of glomerulonephritis mainly concerns nomenclature.

The original term, membranoproliferative glomerulonephritis, has tended to be replaced by the terms mesangiocapillary glomerulonephritis type I and type II. While these two forms of glomerulonephritis were easily confused using older histological techniques, they are clearly separate morphological entities which have little in common apart from the characteristic finding of double contours in peripheral capillary walls.

This section (6.6.5) deals only with membranoproliferative glomerulonephritis (or mesangiocapillary glomerulonephritis type I) which is characterized by subendothelial deposits with varying degrees of mesangial cell interposition and double contours due to reduplication of the basement membrane in peripheral capillary walls. Associated with this capillary wall change there is an increase in mesangial cells and mesangial matrix of variable degree. Figures 6.6.5–1 and 6.6.5–2 illustrate the typical features on light microscopy and electron microscopy. This lesion is illustrated in detail because of the importance of distinguishing the lesions from dense deposit disease which is dealt with in 6.6.6 and which behaves differently in pregnancy.

We first became aware of the potentially serious outcome of pregnancy in patients with membranoproliferative glomerulonephritis or type I mesangiocapillary glomerulonephritis when we encountered a patient with this form of glomerulonephritis in 1961 in whom deterioration occurred abruptly in early pregnancy.

This young woman (EL) whose course has been documented previously (Kincaid-Smith et al 1967), had a renal biopsy a month before she became pregnant. At the time of the biopsy she had mild proteinuria (<1 g/24 h), normal blood pressure and normal renal function and had had a stable course documented over a 2 year period. The renal biopsy showed diffuse membranoproliferative glomerulonephritis (mesangiocapillary type I) with no crescents. The urinary erythrocyte count was high as is usual in this histological category of glomerulonephritis.

At 9 weeks in her first pregnancy she had an acute onset of the nephrotic syndrome and severe hypertension (190/120) and renal function deteriorated rapidly to oliguric renal failure. She died of renal failure 6 weeks later because maintenance dialysis was not available in 1961. A renal biopsy at the time of the oliguric renal failure revealed diffuse crescent formation superimposed

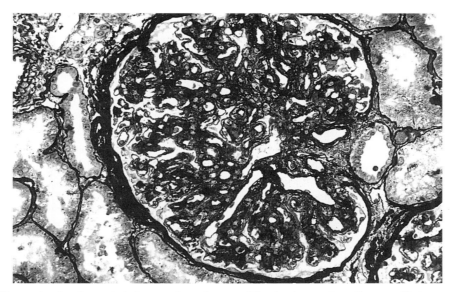

Fig. 6.6.5–1   Glomerulus showing typical changes of membranoproliferative (mesangiocapillary type I) glomerulonephritis.

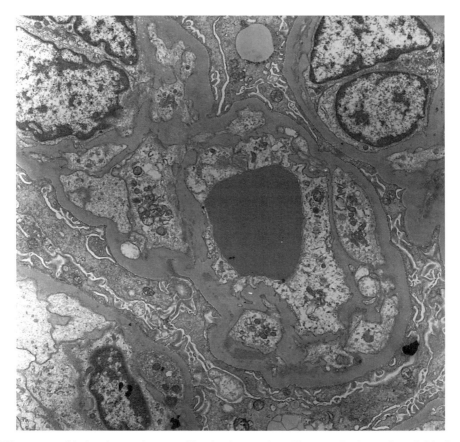

Fig. 6.6.5–2   Ultrastructural lesions in membranoproliferative (mesangiocapillary type I) glomerulonephritis showing double contours and dense subendothelial deposits.

on the previous apparently benign and quiescent glomerular lesion documented only a month before pregnancy. In this patient there appeared to be sound clinical and histological evidence that pregnancy had precipitated acute renal failure accompanied by severe hypertension and the nephrotic syndrome in a patient whose course had previously been stable and in whom normal renal function and an inactive biopsy lesion had been documented just 1 month before pregnancy.

While crescents are seen outside the context of pregnancy in membranoproliferative glomerulonephritis (unlike membranous glomerulonephritis discussed in 6.6.3), the timing of the development of crescents was accurately documented in this patient to coincide with early pregnancy. Crescents have also been documented by us during pregnancy in membranous glomerulonephritis, mesangial IgA glomerulonephritis and lupus glomerulonephritis. Their development adjacent to the subendothelial deposits of preeclampsia in glomerulonephritis suggests that they are related to these subendothelial deposits, and thus to the factors which cause the glomerular lesions of preeclampsia.

Our subsequent experience in this form of glomerulonephritis was documented in 1973 (Fairley et al 1973) (Table 6.6.5–1). Although the number of patients has always been small our results in membranoproliferative glomerulonephritis have been generally worse than other forms of glomerulonephritis (Fairley et al 1973). Of 7 patients with this histological diagnosis only one had a successful pregnancy. Two patients, including the patient documented above, died of renal failure associated with pregnancy. Since that time this form of glomerulonephritis has become very rare in Australia and we have not had the opportunity to study the course of further patients during pregnancy. Our early experience caused us to discourage patients from attempting pregnancy, particularly in view of the unpredictable course illustrated in EL. In our report of pregnancy in glomerulonephritis (Packham et al 1989) the 18 cases included those with dense deposit disease discussed under 6.6.6.

The largest number of pregnancies in patients with membranoproliferative glomerulonephritis was reported by Cameron et al (1983). They

Table 6.6.5–1   Mesangiocapillary glomerulonephritis (from Fairley et al 1973, with permission)

	Pregnancies
Successful pregnancy	
Normal maternal renal function (second pregnancy)	1*
Unsuccessful pregnancy	
Impaired maternal renal function with superimposed preeclamptic toxaemia and neonatal death	1*
Normal maternal renal function but fetal death in utero	1
Impaired maternal renal function that deteriorated further during pregnancy-subsequent death in renal failure	1
Termination of pregnancy at 3 months with normal renal function	2
Termination of pregnancy because of acute deterioration of function at 10 weeks. Maternal death in oliguric renal failure 3 weeks later	1

*Same patient 2 pregnancies.

recorded 20 pregnancies in 7 women which resulted in 8 live births, 5 spontaneous abortions and 7 induced abortions. They did not observe deterioration of renal function during pregnancy. Barcelo et al (1986) from their studies in 16 patients concluded that women with membranoproliferative glomerulonephritis fare worse in pregnancy than those with other lesions. Blood pressure increased in pregnancy in 13 of 16 women and renal function declined in 2. One of these progressed rapidly during and after pregnancy to end stage renal failure. Surian et al (1984) also observed worse results in pregnancy in a small number of patients with membranoproliferative glomerulonephritis.

Rovati et al (1984) in their analysis of the rate of decline of renal function, based on the slope derived from the reciprocal of the creatinine against time, also indicated a worse outcome in pregnancy in membranoproliferative glomerulonephritis. Membranoproliferative glomerulonephritis has become very rare in Western countries over the past 20 years. It remains common in Third World countries and I (PK-S) have recently examined the biopsy and clinical details of a patient from the Philippines in whom the course was very similar to that of EL discussed above. The nephrotic syndrome, severe hypertension and impaired renal function developed in early pregnancy and led to death from renal failure. Another remarkably similar case report appears in a recent report by Badr (1991).

Acute renal failure during pregnancy due to superimposed thrombotic microangiopathy has been recorded in 1 woman with membranoproliferative glomerulonephritis (Perez et al 1988). As this patient is recorded as having focal necrosis of glomeruli in a biopsy during pregnancy and focal necrosis is likely to progress to crescent formation, this may have been an underlying mechanism in EL and in Badr's case.

General experience suggests that this form of glomerulonephritis is usually associated with a poor outcome of pregnancy for both mother and fetus although the experience of Cameron et al (1983) was rather better than that of other groups.

REFERENCES

Badr K F 1991 Arachidonate cyclo-oxygenase and lipoxygenase products in the mediation of glomerular immune injury. Nephrology, Dialysis, Transplantation 6: 662–669

Barcelo P, Lopez-Lillo J, Cabero L et al 1986 Successful pregnancy in primary glomerular disease. Kidney International 30: 914–919

Cameron J W, Turner D R, Heaton J et al 1983 Idiopathic mesangiocapillary glomerulonephritis. American Journal of Medicine 74: 175–192

Fairley K F, Whitworth J A, Kincaid-Smith P 1973 Glomerulonephritis and pregnancy. In: P Kincaid-Smith, T H Mathew, E L Becker (eds) Glomerulonephritis. Wiley, New York, p 697

Kincaid-Smith P, Fairley K F, Bullen L 1967 Kidney disease and pregnancy. Medical Journal of Australia 2: 1155–1159

Packham D K, North R A, Fairley K F et al 1989 Primary glomerulonephritis and pregnancy. Quarterly Journal of Medicine 70: 537–553

Perez A J, Sobrado S, Courel M et al 1988 Renal thrombotic microangiopathy in a pregnant patient with membranoproliferative glomerulonephritis. Nephron 49: 86–87

Rovati C, Perrino M L, Barbiano di Belgiojoso G et al 1984 Pregnancy and course of primary glomerulonephritis. Contributions to Nephrology 37: 182–189

Surian M, Imbasciati E, Cosci P et al 1984 Glomerular disease and pregnancy. Nephron 36: 101–105

6.6.6 Dense deposit disease (mesangiocapillary glomerulonephritis type II)

Now that the morphological lesion in dense deposit disease (Figs. 6.6.6–1 and 6.6.6–2) can be clearly differentiated from that of membranoproliferative glomerulonephritis with subendothelial deposits, the pregnancy outcome in these two distinct morphological categories should be considered separately and appears to be different. The light and electron microscopy are illustrated because of the past confusion between these lesions and those illustrated in Figures 6.6.5–1 and 6.6.5–2.

We have been able to find very little documentation of the outcome in pregnancy in series of patients with dense deposit disease. Cameron et al (1983) reported 9 pregnancies in women with 'active' disease; 5 of these pregnancies occurred in 1 patient resulting in 2 live births and 3 terminations. They recorded no deterioration of renal function during pregnancy.

Our own experience in 14 pregnancies in 7 patients with dense deposit disease has indicated a more benign course than that seen in membranoproliferative glomerulonephritis (mesangiocapillary glomerulonephritis type I) (Bennett et al 1989); 4 patients presented for the first time during pregnancy and the diagnosis was made at that time. As indicated in other sections of this book, presentation during pregnancy with complications of pregnancy is generally associated with a worse outcome but this was not obvious in this group of patients. Both proteinuria and hypertension were present in all pregnancies but renal function did not deteriorate.

All women had live babies and only 1 was premature.

We found no evidence in this group of patients of an adverse effect of pregnancy on the course of the glomerulonephritis. It should be recognized, however, that all the women who had pregnancies belonged to the more benign category of patients with dense deposit disease, which we have identified.

In a study of 27 patients with dense deposit disease we identified two groups of patients: one group ran a stable course but in the other, renal function deteriorated. The characteristic findings in those in whom deterioration occurred were recurrent macroscopic haematuria, high urinary erythrocyte count, heavy proteinuria and high urinary leucocyte count. All these features were significantly different when those with a good prognosis were compared with those who progressed.

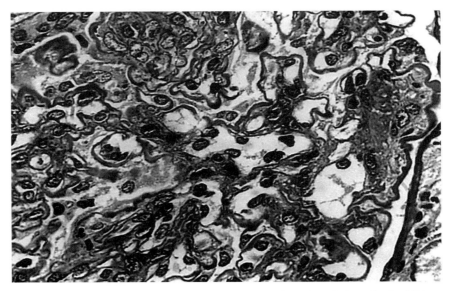

Fig. 6.6.6–1 Glomerulus from a patient with dense deposit disease. The 'dense deposits' are clearly visible as a dark wavy line on the outer border of all glomerular capillaries.

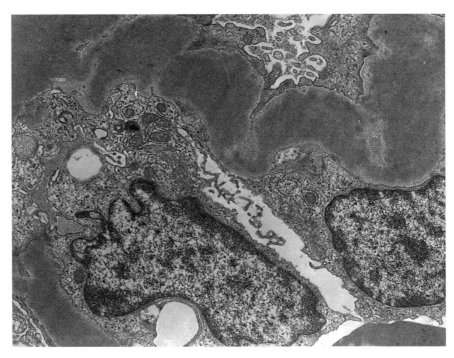

Fig. 6.6.6–2 Ultrastructure in dense deposit disease in which the basement membrane is virtually replaced by electron dense deposits.

Renal function remained stable in the patients without the above clinical features. All the pregnancies which we observed occurred in the stable group whom we identified as having a better prognosis.

Although few data are available on series of patients with dense deposit disease in pregnancy, there are a number of individual reports of acute deterioration related to pregnancy. Montoliu et al (1982) reported the course of a patient in whom acute renal failure developed in association with crescent formation and in whom plasma exchange resulted in recovery of renal function.

Leichter et al (1986) reported a very similar case with crescents in 51% of glomeruli which developed in the postpartum period and resulted in end stage renal failure.

Another single case with a good long term outcome was reported by Inaba et al (1989).

In most reports of membranoproliferative or mesangiocapillary glomerulonephritis in pregnancy, the distinction between type I and type II lesions or dense deposit disease is not made (Klockers et al 1980, Strauch & Hayslett 1974, Surian et al 1984, Jungers et al 1986).

In general, however, a poor outcome in pregnancy is documented in patients with membranoproliferative glomerulonephritis but this has not been our experience in dense deposit disease. Clearly, from the cases reported by Montoliu et al (1982) and Leichter et al (1986) severe acute deterioration of renal function may occur in the mother in association with crescent formation. It is likely from the clinical features documented by Montoliu and by Leichter that the patients in whom they described acute deterioration of renal function belonged to the progressive group characterized by recurrent macroscopic haematuria, heavy proteinuria and heavy continuing microscopic haematuria.

It may therefore be particularly important when counselling patients with dense deposit disease who wish to undertake pregnancy to bear in mind that a low urine protein level, low urinary erythrocyte and leucocyte count, absence of nephrotic syndrome and macroscopic haematuria are the features likely to be associated with a satisfactory outcome in pregnancy. Both a high urinary erythrocyte count and a high urinary leucocyte count are likely to be associated with crescent formation on biopsy (Segasothy et al 1989).

REFERENCES

Bennett W M, Fassett R G, Walker R G et al 1989 Mesangiocapillary glomerulonephritis type II (dense deposit disease): clinical features of progressive disease. American Journal of Kidney Diseases 13: 469–476

Cameron S J, Turner D R, Heaton J et al 1983 Idiopathic mesangiocapillary glomerulonephritis. American Journal of Medicine 74: 175–192

Inaba S, Tanizawa T, Igarashi T et al 1989 Long-term follow-up of membranoproliferative glomerulonephritis type II and pregnancy: a case report. Clinical Nephrology 32: 10–13

Jungers P, Forget D, Henry-Amar M et al 1986 Chronic kidney disease and pregnancy. Advances in Nephrology 15: 103–141

Klockers M, Saarikoski S, Ikonen E et al 1980 Pregnancy in patients with renal disease. Acta Medica Scandinavica 207: 207–214

Leichter H E, Jordan S C, Cohen A H et al 1986 Postpartum renal failure in a patient with membranoproliferative glomerulonephritis Type II. American Journal of Nephrology 6: 382–385

Montoliu J, Bergada E, Arrizabalaga P et al 1982 Acute renal failure in dense deposit disease: recovery after plasmapheresis. British Medical Journal 284: 940

Segasothy M, Fairley K F, Birch D F et al 1989 Immunoperoxidase identification of nucleated cells in the urine in glomerular disease and acute tubular disorders. Clinical Nephrology 31: 286–291

Strauch B S, Hayslett J P 1974 Kidney disease and pregnancy. British Medical Journal 7: 578–582

Surian M, Imbasciati E, Banfi G et al 1984 Glomerular disease and pregnancy. Nephron 36: 101–105

6.6.7 Endocapillary glomerulonephritis (postinfectious and poststreptococcal glomerulonephritis)

This histological category of glomerulonephritis is characterized by large cellular glomeruli in which there is significant endocapillary proliferation accompanied by infiltration by polymorphonuclear leucocytes and mononuclear leucocytes and macrophages (Fig. 6.6.7–1). On immunoperoxidase or immunofluorescent staining prominent C3 staining of extramembranous deposits is characteristic; on electron microscopy these deposits appear as subepithelial humps.

This histological form of glomerulonephritis most commonly occurs some 10 days after an infective illness, the infection being most

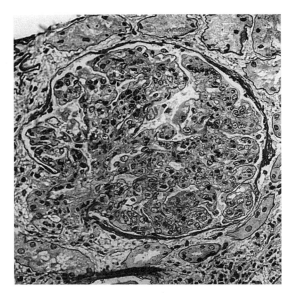

Fig. 6.6.7–1   Glomerulus from a patient with endocapillary glomerulonephritis showing a great increase in cells, including many polymorphs as the major abnormality.

frequently due to so-called nephritogenic strains of streptococci.

Clinically this event is accompanied by oedema, hypertension, impairment of renal function, oliguria and macroscopic haematuria. Most useful confirmatory tests, apart from renal biopsy, are a low serum complement and rising antistreptolysin titre.

Acute glomerulonephritis occurring during pregnancy is rare and it is probably less prevalent now in developed countries than it was in the past. The only 2 clearly documented cases which we have seen occurred 25 years ago (Kincaid-Smith et al 1967) and in spite of a large referral of patients with renal disease in pregnancy we have not encountered subsequent cases.

Nadler et al (1969) who described a patient with acute glomerulonephritis during pregnancy drew attention to the fact that acute glomerulonephritis had not been documented in over 15 000 deliveries at the Jewish General Hospital in Montreal (Sabin et al 1960) or in 36 years at the Sloane Hospital (Kaplan et al 1962). Nadler et al (1969) were able to find only 19 women with acute glomerulonephritis in pregnancy described in the literature and only the 2 which

we described were documented histologically as endocapillary glomerulonephritis (Kincaid-Smith et al 1967). Renal biopsy was not performed in the other cases reviewed by Nadler et al (1969).

Fetal outcome in the cases reviewed by Nadler et al (1969) appeared to be related to hypertension. If the diastolic blood pressure was over 110 mmHg the pregnancy was either terminated or fetal death occurred in utero. When the diastolic blood pressure was below 100 mmHg, 6 of 8 pregnancies had a successful outcome.

More recently, Fukuda et al (1988) reported a case proven on renal biopsy in which the pregnancy was successful in spite of a severe nephrotic syndrome developing between 31 and 34 weeks' gestation.

REFERENCES

Fukuda O, Ito M, Nakayama M et al 1988 Acute glomerulonephritis during the third trimester of pregnancy. International Journal of Gynaecology and Obstetrics 26: 141–144
Kaplan A L, Smith J P, Tillman A J B 1962 Healed acute and chronic nephritis in pregnancy. American Journal of Obstetrics and Gynecology 83: 1519
Kincaid-Smith P, Fairley K F, Bullen M 1967 Kidney disease and pregnancy. Medical Journal of Australia 2: 1155–1159
Nadler N, Salinas-Madrigal L, Charles A G et al 1969 Acute glomerulonephritis during late pregnancy. Obstetrics and Gynecology 34:277–283
Sabin M, Parliament D, Strean G J 1960 A ten year review of renal disease in pregnancy. Canadian Medical Association Journal 83:372

6.6.8   An overview of pregnancy in patients with glomerulonephritis

When nephrology first began to emerge as a specialty and when nephrologists started to be consulted about pregnancy in women with renal disease, the conservative view of the obstetrician (Browne & Browne 1960) about the outcome of pregnancy in women with renal disease came under challenge. Addis (1949) and Goldring & Chassis (1964) questioned whether pregnancy or the superimposed hypertension which developed in pregnancy aggravated the underlying renal disease. Browne's view was based on a study by Dodds & Browne (1940) in which the outcome of 21 pregnancies in 17 patients with glomerulonephritis was documented. Although 62% of pregnancies produced living infants, 8 of 17 mothers died or developed terminal uraemia 6 months to 12 years later. Dodds & Browne advised that 'termination of pregnancy as soon as the condition is diagnosed was usually the best treatment from the point of view of the mother's expectation of life'. Hamilton (1952) studied all women with nephritis complicating pregnancy over a 10 year period at the Simpson Memorial Maternity Hospital and observed deterioration in the mother in 89% of cases and fetal loss in 72%.

Browne & Browne (1960) gave very clear advice in the case of women with impaired renal function — 'There can be no doubt that if the blood urea is above 40 mg% the pregnancy should be terminated at once' — and subsequent experience tended to support this view. Our early experience in 11 pregnancies in 9 patients with urea levels over 50 mg/100 ml helped to confirm a gloomy outlook for the mother if renal function is impaired (Kincaid-Smith et al 1967). Although careful management of hypertension and other maternal complications permitted a successful outcome in 9 of the 11 pregnancies, in the women whom we studied urea levels rose during pregnancy in every case and in only 1 patient did the level fall again after pregnancy; 5 patients showed serious rapid deterioration during pregnancy, and 3 of these patients died and 2 required maintenance dialysis after the pregnancy. These patients clearly deteriorated more rapidly during pregnancy than would have been anticipated as part of the natural history of the underlying renal disease. It is now generally accepted that women with impaired renal function run a significant risk of accelerated deterioration during pregnancy (Becker et al 1985, Hou et al 1985). In 1967 we found that all 23 patients with relatively mild glomerular lesions had successful pregnancies; however, 20% of cases with more severe glomerular lesions sustained fetal loss. A small number of patients, however, with inactive biopsies, progressed rapidly to renal failure. The stable course and normal renal function, inactive renal biopsy appearances and absence of hypertension in 2 patients who progressed rapidly to renal failure demonstrated to us that it was difficult to predict which patients may suffer deterioration in renal function during pregnancy. Crescent formation was noted on biopsies in 2 patients who deteriorated (Kincaid-Smith et al 1967), and the development of crescents during pregnancy is one mechanism whereby deterioration in renal function may occur in patients with glomerulonephritis (Fairley et al 1973, Fairley & Packham 1989).

The other histological lesion which closely resembles preeclampsia (Kincaid-Smith & Fairley 1987) and which occurs as a superimposed segmental lesion in patients with glomerulonephritis is that of focal and segmental hyalinosis.

Although we have reported this as a complication of pregnancy in several forms of glomerulonephritis, we have been able to document its occurrence most accurately in mesangial IgA glomerulonephritis.

Segmental hyalinosis occurs in only 8.9% of biopsies from women with mesangial IgA glomerulonephritis who are not pregnant but in 58% of biopsies taken during pregnancy or in the early postpartum period (Table 6.6.2–4). This glomerular lesion may contribute to the irreversible deterioration of renal function and increased proteinuria seen in some cases of glomerulonephritis.

One of the difficulties in assessing the likely outcome in the individual patient with glomerulonephritis is the paucity of studies dealing with any particular form of glomerulonephritis during pregnancy. In 6.6.1–6.6.7 such data, as are available, in the different morphological forms of glomerulonephritis are reviewed.

Our overall experience in 395 pregnancies in women with glomerulonephritis (Packham et al 1989) shows that fetal loss occurs in 26% of pregnancies, 5% being therapeutic abortions. Prematurity occurs in 24% of cases and 15% are small for gestational age. Perinatal mortality is also common (14%). As far as the maternal outcome is concerned, the three major risk factors for progression in glomerulonephritis — namely, proteinuria, hypertension and renal function — may all be adversely affected by pregnancy. Of these, potentially the most serious is the deterioration in renal function which was documented in 15% of pregnancies and which failed to resolve in the postpartum period in 5%. Proteinuria, another well documented risk factor for progression in glomerulonephritis, increased in almost 60% of pregnancies in women with glomerulonephritis and this increased proteinuria failed to resolve after pregnancy in 15%.

Hypertension, the third major risk factor for progression in glomerulonephritis, developed during pregnancy in 40% of cases. It had an early onset in pregnancy in 26% and was severe in 18%. Of women who developed hypertension 'de novo' during pregnancy, 18% showed persisting hypertension 6 months after the pregnancy.

Thus, at the end of pregnancy in this large series of cases, 5% of women had suffered irreversible deterioration in renal function, 15% had developed an irreversible increase in proteinuria and 18% developed de novo hypertension in pregnancy which persisted after pregnancy.

This is perhaps the most clear cut evidence that pregnancy may alter the course of renal disease. Hypertension, the degree of proteinuria and impaired renal function are the three major risk factors for progression of all forms of glomerular disease in which this relationship has been studied. It appears from this that the patients who, at the end of a pregnancy have worse renal function, heavier proteinuria and have developed hypertension, are at greater risk of subsequent deterioration from their glomerulonephritis than they were before the pregnancy. Although this has been a point of controversy and disagreement, there are, nonetheless, overwhelming data to suggest that hypertension impaired renal function and the degree of proteinuria are the major risk factors for progression in glomerulonephritis.

There are only a very small number of studies documenting the course of and outcome of pregnancy in large series of women with glomerulonephritis. Our own study of 395 pregnancies in 238 women with biopsy proven glomerulonephritis is the largest. Katz et al (1980) studied 81 pregnancies in 54 women, Surian et al (1984) studied 114 pregnancies in 80 women and Jungers et al (1986) 240 pregnancies in 122 women. The results in these studies are overall remarkably similar in terms of fetal loss and maternal outcome (Table 6.6.8–1), which is perhaps surprising in view of the different ways in which the data were collected. The studies by Katz et al

(1980), Surian et al (1984), and Jungers et al (1986) were retrospective analyses of the outcome in women with renal disease in whom data were available relating to previous pregnancies. In only 141 of the 395 pregnancies which we recorded were the data derived retrospectively. In 254 pregnancies the patient presented to us during pregnancy, hence the biopsy diagnosis was obtained after the commencement of pregnancy. Because these patients were referred with a pregnancy related complication, one might assume that the outcome of pregnancy for fetus and mother might be worse in the group presenting during pregnancy. Maternal outcome details are given in Table 6.6.8–2; both hypertension and increased proteinuria were more frequent in the patients presenting during pregnancy as were overall adverse maternal events.

Fetal loss beyond 20 weeks gestation was 20% significantly higher in women presenting during pregnancy than in those in whom the pregnancy occurred after the diagnosis was known, in whom it was 5% (Packham et al 1989).

Although it has been claimed by some that our results in pregnancy in patients with glomerulonephritis are less good than those reported from elsewhere, Table 6.6.8–1 shows that our results differ little from those of other studies. The area where we do differ is in the interpretation of those results. In Table 6.6.8–1 it will be seen that 4–28% of patients reported in that larger series progressed to end stage renal disease within the study period while only 6% of our own patients progressed. In spite of this low figure, we believe that we have evidence from careful studies of individual patients that some suffered irreversible deterioration which we could attribute to the pregnancy. We discuss these in detail in 6.6.1–6.6.7. An example of this is seen in the appearance of crescents on biopsy in 3 patients with membranous glomerulonephritis during pregnancy. Crescents are an extremely uncommon finding in membranous glomerulonephritis. In over 30 years in a very large number of serial biopsies in patients with membranous glomerulonephritis we have only seen crescents on biopsy in these 3 women and in 1 other patient. The fourth was a man who developed postinfectious glomerulonephritis superimposed on membranous

Table 6.6.8–1 Comparison of published series of pregnancies in patients with primary glomerulonephritis (from Packham et al 1989, with permission)

	Katz et al 1980 (n = 54, 81 pregnancies 83 fetuses)		Surian et al 1984 (n = 80, 114 pregnancies 114 fetuses)		Jungers et al 1986 (n = 122, 240 pregnancies 244 fetuses)		Our series (n = 238, 395 pregnancies 398 fetuses)	
	No	%	No.	%	No.	%	No.	%
Fetal outcome								
Therapeutic abortions	–		–		49	20	22	6
Spontaneous abortions	–						22	6
Stillbirths	5	6	17	15	13	5	34	8
Neonatal deaths	5	6					24	6
Total fetal loss	10	12	17	15	62	25	102	26
Premature (live)	16	19	14	12	29	12	95	24
Small for gestational age	21	25	6	5	20	12	36	15
Maternal outcome								
Impaired renal function								
Irreversible			3	3	–		11	3
Reversible			6	5			49	12
Total	14	17	9	8	17	7	60	15
Hypertension								
Irreversible	–		10	9	–		44	11
Reversible	–		13	11	–		135	34
Exacerbation	–		–		–		28	7
Total	37	46	23	20	80	33	207	52
Severe	18	22	–		–		71	18
Increased proteinuria								
Irreversible	18	22	–		–		35	9
Reversible	30	37	–		–		196	50
Total	48	59	–		58	24	231	59
Chronic renal failure/end state renal disease at end of study period	8	15	3	4	34	28	14	6

glomerulonephritis and this occurrence was accompanied by diffuse crescent formation (Kincaid-Smith 1975). It seems clear to us, therefore, that crescents developing in patients with membranous glomerulonephritis during pregnancy cannot be regarded as part of the natural history of membranous glomerulonephritis but must represent an adverse effect of pregnancy. We were able to demonstrate (Fairley et al 1973) that crescents developed adjacent to the subendothelial deposits of preeclampsia linking crescent formation to this specific glomerular lesion which is seen only during pregnancy in patients with preeclampsia. The development of crescents clearly influenced the course of the disease being accompanied by increase in proteinuria, severe hypertension and deterioration in renal function (Kincaid-Smith 1975) (Fig. 6.6.3–3). The fact that a very mild membranous lesion progressed to destruction of 75% of glomeruli by crescent formation during pregnancy in the patient illustrated in Figure 6.6.3–3 is, to us, compelling evidence that pregnancy was a contributing factor in the deterioration observed in that patient. Such detailed studies of individual patients, some of whom were followed by us for up to 30 years, leave us in no doubt that, in individual cases, pregnancy has an adverse effect on renal disease.

Because of its usually very benign course, particularly in women (Murphy et al 1988), membranous glomerulonephritis provides a very good model for the study of the influence of pregnancy on glomerular disease.

We would find the results published by Studd & Blainey (1969) for pregnancy in membranous glomerulonephritis very disappointing indeed; 2

Table 6.6.8–2   Comparison of maternal outcome of pregnancies pre and post diagnosis (from Packham et al 1989, with permission)

Maternal outcome	Before diagnosis ($n = 254$)			After diagnosis ($n = 141$)	
	No.	%		No.	%
Impaired renal function					
Irreversible	9	3		2	1
Reversible	37	15		12	9
Total	46	18	NS	14	10
Hypertension					
Irreversible	33	13		11	18
Reversible	119	47		16	11
Exacerbation	9	4		19	13
Total	161	64	$P<0.005$	46	32
Early	84	33	$P<0.005$	20	14
Severe	59	23	$P<0.005$	12	9
Increased proteinuria					
Irreversible	30	12		5	4
Reversible	138	54		58	41
Total	168	66	$P<0.005$	63	45
Stable proteinuria	25	10		31	22

of the 5 young women with membranous glomerulonephritis died of malignant hypertension — something quite outside our experience of this disease based on a long term study of the natural history of membranous glomerulonephritis in 62 women (Murphy et al 1988). Of the 5 women in Studd & Blainey's series 3 had diastolic blood pressures during pregnancy of 120–130 mmHg and in 2 of the 3 this developed during pregnancy. Surely this must be interpreted as evidence of an adverse effect of pregnancy on the underlying membranous glomerulonephritis. Severe hypertension is a rare finding in membranous glomerulonephritis (Murphy et al 1988).

The fact that crescents developed at the site of typical subendothelial deposits of preeclampsia (Fairley et al 1973) leaves us in little doubt that the crescents developing in pregnancy in patients with membranous glomerulonephritis are the result of superimposed preeclampsia.

Cameron & Hicks (1984) in a review of this topic reported deterioration in renal function in 6–18% of the different forms of glomerulonephritis which was irreversible in 50% of the cases in which renal function deteriorated (Table 6.6.8–3).

Rovati et al (1984), in an analysis of the slope of the reciprocal of the serum creatinine in 29 patients with glomerulonephritis who had normal renal function at the beginning of the study, found that pregnancy had an adverse effect in focal and segmental hyalinosis sclerosis (8 cases) and membranoproliferative glomerulonephritis (5 cases) but not in Berger's disease (11 cases).

The most clear cut factor which influences the outcome of pregnancy in patients with glomerulonephritis is impaired renal function and it is now generally agreed, as reported from Melbourne in early studies (Mackay 1963, Kincaid-Smith et al 1967), that a raised serum creatinine is likely to be associated with deterioration in renal function during pregnancy (Becker et al 1985, Hou et al 1985).

The nephrotic syndrome has been identified by Jungers et al (1991) as an independent risk factor for a poor fetal outcome. It was also associated with a poor fetal and maternal outcome in our patients with membranous glomerulonephritis in pregnancy (Packham et al 1987b).

Controversy exists with regard to the influence of preexisting hypertension on pregnancy in patients with glomerulonephritis. Several authors state that hypertension has adverse effects for mother and fetus (Bear 1976, Katz & Lindheimer 1985, Imbasciati et al 1986, Jungers et al 1986). In our own study of 105 pregnancies in 76 women (55 normotensive, 21 hypertensive) apart from

Table 6.6.8–3 Pregnancy in glomerulonephritis (from Becker et al 1985 with permission; originally from Cameron & Hicks 1984)

| | No. of pregnancies | No. of patients | Deterioration in renal function | | Pregnancies (%) | Patients (%) |
			Reversible	Irreversible		
FSGS	39	28	2	3	13	18
MCGN	58	37*	2	1	8	14
Membranous	72	54	2	1	4	7
IgA	52	34	2	0	4	6
'Focal'	27	13	4	0	4	8
'Proliferative'	45	34	4	2	9	12

FSGS, focal and segmental glomerular sclerosis; MCGN, mesangiocapillary glomerulonephritis.

smaller babies in the hypertensive group we were unable to find adverse effects in women who were hypertensive prior to pregnancy. The only difference between the two groups was that patients with preexisting hypertension were more likely to have a high blood pressure recorded in early pregnancy, a not surprising finding (Packham et al 1987a). The development of severe hypertension in pregnancy had more serious consequences in the period when only a few antihypertensive agents were available. The very bad outcome in Studd & Blainey's (1969) patients who developed severe hypertension in pregnancy, 2 of whom died of malignant hypertension, would presumably not occur at the present time.

In summary, therefore, although the majority of patients with glomerulonephritis can achieve a successful pregnancy without any great risk of deterioration in function, a few cases suffer adverse effects during pregnancy and this cannot always be predicted with any accuracy except in the case of patients with impaired renal function where the likelihood of further deterioration during pregnancy is very high.

REFERENCES

Addis 1949 Glomerular nephritis: diagnosis and treatment. Mac Millan, New York
Bear R 1976 Pregnancy in patients with renal disease: a study of 44 cases. Obstetrics and Gynecology 48: 13–18
Becker G, Fairley K F, Whitworth J A 1985 Pregnancy exacerbates glomerular disease. American Journal of Kidney Diseases 4: 266–272
Browne F J, Browne JCMc 1960 Antenatal and postnatal care, 9th edn. Churchill Livingstone, London
Cameron J S, Hicks J 1984 Pregnancy in patients with pre-existing glomerular disease. Contributions Nephrology 37: 149–156
Dodds G H, Browne F J 1940 Chronic nephritis in pregnancy. Proceedings of the Royal Society of Medicine: Section of Obstetrics and Gynaecology 33: 737–740
Fairley C K, Packham D K 1989 Glomerular crescents and pregnancy. American Journal of Kidney Diseases 13: 250–252
Fairley K F, Whitworth J A, Kincaid-Smith P 1973 Glomerulonephritis and pregnancy In: P Kincaid-Smith, T H Mathew, E L Becker (eds) Glomerulonephritis. Wiley, New York, 997–1011
Goldring C, Chassis H 1964 Hypertension and hypertensive disease. Commonwealth Fund, New York
Hamilton F H 1952 Nephritis in pregnancy: a follow-up study. Journal of Obstetrics and Gynaecology 59: 25–29
Hou S, Grossman S, Madias N 1985 Pregnancy in women with renal disease and moderate renal insufficiency. American Journal of Medicine 78: 185–194
Imbasciati E, Pardi G, Gapetta P et al 1986 Pregnancy in women with chronic renal failure. American Journal of Nephrology 61: 193–198
Jungers P, Forget D, Henry-Amar M et al 1986 Chronic kidney disease and pregnancy. Advances in Nephrology 15: 103–141
Jungers P, Houillier P, Forget D et al 1991 Specific controversies concerning the natural history of renal disease in pregnancy. American Journal of Kidney Diseases 17: 116–122
Katz A I, Lindheimer M D 1985 Does pregnancy aggravate primary glomerular disease? American Journal of Kidney Diseases 6: 261–272
Katz A I, Davison J M, Hayslett J P et al 1980 Pregnancy in women with kidney disease. Kidney International 18: 192–206
Kincaid-Smith P (ed) 1975 The kidney — a clinicopathological study. Blackwell Scientific, Oxford
Kincaid-Smith P, Fairley K F, Bullen M 1967 Kidney disease and pregnancy. Medical Journal of Australia 2: 1155–1159
Kincaid-Smith P, Fairley K F 1987 Renal disease in pregnancy. Three controversial areas: mesangial IgA nephropathy, focal glomerular sclerosis (focal and segmental hyalinosis and sclerosis), and reflux nephropathy. American Journal of Kidney Diseases 9: 328–333
Mackay E V 1963 Pregnancy and renal disease: a ten year survey. Australian and New Zealand Journal of Obstetrics and Gynecology 3: 21–24

Murphy B F, Fairley K F, Kincaid-Smith P 1988 Idiopathic
    membranous glomerulonephritis: long-term follow-up in
    139 cases. Clinical Nephrology 30: 175–181
Packham D K, Fairley K F, Ihle B U et al 1987a Comparison
    of pregnancy outcome between normotensive and
    hypertensive women with primary glomerulonephritis.
    Clinical and Experimental Hypertension B6(3): 387–399
Packham D K, North R A, Fairley K F et al 1987b
    Membranous glomerulonephritis and pregnancy. Clinical
    Nephrology 28: 56–64
Packham D K, North R A, Fairley K F et al 1989 Primary
    glomerulonephritis and pregnancy. Quarterly Journal of
    Medicine 266: 537–553
Rovati C, Perrino M L, Barbiano di Belgiojoso G et al 1984
    Pregnancy and course of primary glomerulonephritis.
    Contributions to Nephrology 37: 182–189
Studd J W, Blainey J D 1969 Pregnancy and the nephrotic
    syndrome. British Medical Journal 1: 276–280
Surian M, Imbasciati E, Cosci P et al 1984 Glomerular
    disease and pregnancy. Study of 123 pregnancies in
    patients with primary and secondary glomerular diseases.
    Nephron 36: 101–105

6.7 GLOMERULONEPHRITIS ASSOCIATED WITH SYSTEMIC DISEASE

6.7.1 Lupus glomerulonephritis

Views on the advisability of pregnancy in patients with lupus glomerulonephritis are surprisingly variable.

On the one hand we have the view of Bear (1976, 1978) that patients with systemic lupus erythematosus active or inactive with or without nephritis should avoid pregnancy. This view was based on a review of the literature at that time and experience in 6 patients, 5 of whom showed an increase in proteinuria which was in the nephrotic range. In 3, the proteinuria persisted in spite of treatment and 2 of these 3 died within 2 years of delivery. A third patient developed malignant hypertension during pregnancy and died of a cerebrovascular accident 2 years later. It is not surprising that this report of a 50% mortality within 2 years of pregnancy in young women should lead Bear to the conclusion that pregnancy should be avoided in patients with lupus glomerulonephritis.

In contrast, Mintz & Rodriquez-Alvarez (1989), on the basis of 58 pregnancies in women with lupus nephritis, conclude that the short term prognosis is good and there is no long term deleterious influence of pregnancy on the evolution of systemic lupus erythematosus.

We have analysed our experience in 64 pregnancies in 41 women with biopsy proven lupus nephritis studied between 1965 and 1991. The methods and definitions used in this study were similar to those outlined in 6.6. All women were under our direct care during pregnancy and the data were accumulated prospectively over the 25 year period.

The fetal outcome is shown in Table 6.7.1–1. The total fetal loss was 22 (34%) including 8 therapeutic and 5 spontaneous abortions. There were 7 stillbirths, all of them in women with a circulating lupus anticoagulant; 4 of these women had impaired renal function and 5 had early hypertension which was severe in 2; 5 showed increase proteinuria; 2 women, who had stillbirths, showed no associated complications.

Among women in whom a neonatal death occurred, 2 of 5 were lupus anticoagulant positive; 2 had impaired renal function and all 5 had early hypertension which was severe in 4; 4 showed an increase in proteinuria which was in the nephrotic range in 2.

Prematurity was recorded in 19 infants (30%) and 5 (8%) were severely premature.

Birth weights were available for 25 infants, 3 were below the 10th percentile for the Australian population.

The influence of presentation during pregnancy on the fetus is shown in Table 6.7.1–2.

In each category in Table 6.7.1–2, the patients whose pregnancy preceded the renal biopsy (patients who presented during pregnancy) had a worse outcome than those in whom the diagnosis was known at the beginning of pregnancy.

Table 6.7.1–1 Fetal outcome ($n = 65$) of pregnancy in women with systemic lupus erythematosus (from Packham et al 1992, with permission)

	No.	%
Spontaneous abortions	5	8
Therapeutic abortions	5	8
Stillbirths	7	11
Neonatal deaths	5	8
Total fetal loss	22	34
Severe prematurity	5	8
Prematurity	14	22
Term	24	37

Table 6.7.1–2 Fetal outcome (from Packham et al 1992, with permission)

	Pregnancy prior to biopsy diagnosis (n = 18)		Pregnancy after biopsy diagnosis (n = 47)	
	No.	%	No.	%
Fetal loss	8	44	14	30
Perinatal mortality	6	33	6	13
Prematurity	6	33	13	22
Live infant at term	4	22	20	42

Table 6.7.1–3 illustrates the serious effects of a circulating lupus anticoagulant on the fetal outcome. Fetal loss was 57% in patients who had a circulating lupus anticoagulant but only 23% in those with no lupus anticoagulant and, as outlined above, all the stillbirths occurred in the lupus anticoagulant positive group.

Women who were lupus anticoagulant negative and in whom pregnancy was undertaken after the biopsy diagnosis had been made, are a selected group in whom a good fetal outcome may be expected. Although overall fetal loss in this group of 34 was 24%, perinatal mortality was only 6%.

The histological lesion on renal biopsy appeared to influence the perinatal mortality. There was no perinatal mortality in women with a membranous lupus glomerulonephritis on renal biopsy, whereas

a perinatal mortality of 24% was recorded in women with a diffuse proliferative glomerulonephritis (P<0.03).

There were no maternal deaths and no patient progressed to end stage renal failure in spite of a follow up period as long as 26 years in some patients. This is in accord with our overall experience of lupus nephritis which generally responds well to treatment and very rarely progresses to end stage renal disease in patients who attend regularly and take the treatment recommended (Leaker et al 1987).

Overall maternal outcome is shown in Table 6.7.1–4. As in the case of fetal outcome the maternal outcome was worse in patients who presented during pregnancy with complications of pregnancy. This is detailed in Table 6.7.1–5.

Impairment of renal function, hypertension and increased proteinuria were all more likely to occur during pregnancy in patients presenting with a complication of pregnancy in whom the biopsy was carried out during or after pregnancy.

Total hypertension, severe hypertension, early hypertension and increased proteinuria were all significantly more frequent in patients who presented with a complication of pregnancy.

The maternal outcome was not different in women who tested positive for a lupus anti-

Table 6.7.1–3 Comparison of fetal outcome of lupus anticoagulant (LAC) positive and negative mothers (from Packham et al 1992, with permission)

Fetal outcome	LAC +ve (n = 21)		LAC −ve (n = 44)	
	No.	%	No.	%
Therapeutic abortion	1	5	4	9
Spontaneous abortion	2	10	3	7
Stillbirth	7	33	0	
Neonatal death	2	10	3	7
Total fetal loss	12*	58	10*	23
Severe premature	0		5	11
Premature	4	19	10	23
Full term	5	24	13	43
Total live births	9**	43	34**	77

*P<0.01, **P<0.001.

Table 6.7.1–4 Maternal outcome in lupus nephritis

	No.	%
Total pregnancies	64	
Impaired renal function		
Irreversible	1	
Reversible	11	
Total	12	19
Hypertension		
Irreversible	9	14
Reversible	19	
Exacerbation	4	6
Total	28	44
Early	18	28
Severe	8	13
Increased proteinuria		
Irreversible	3	5
Reversible	28	44
Total	31	
Nephrotic	11	17

Table 6.7.1–5   Comparison of maternal outcome of pregnancies which occurred before and after diagnosis (from Packham et al 1992, with permission)

Maternal outcome	Before biopsy diagnosis (n = 18)			After biopsy diagnosis (n = 46)	
	No.	%		No.	%
Impaired renal function					
Irreversible	1	5		0	–
Reversible	5	28		6	13
Total	6	33	NS	6	13
Hypertension					
Irreversible	6	33		3	7
Reversible	8	44		7	15
Exacerbation	0	–		4	9
Total	14	78	P = 0.0016	14	30
Early	9	50	P = 0.033	9	20
Severe	6	33	P = 0.008	2	4
Increased proteinuria					
Irreversible	2	11		1	2
Reversible	13	72		15	33
Total	15	83	P = 0.0013	16	35

coagulant from those with a negative lupus anticoagulant test (Table 6.7.1–6).

Impairment of renal function was recorded in 33% of lupus anticoagulant positive and 12% of lupus anticoagulant negative women but this was not statistically significant. This is surprising in view of the frequency with which we recorded acute vascular lesions on biopsy in pregnancy in women with a lupus anticoagulant (Kincaid-Smith et al 1988).

Histological lesions on biopsy also surprisingly had no effect on maternal outcome (Packham et al 1992).

This may reflect the fact that the majority of pregnancies took place after the renal lesion had been treated. We expect and often achieve a remarkable degree of histological resolution of diffuse and focal proliferative lupus lesions (Kincaid-Smith 1967, Leaker et al 1987).

In several cases pregnancies occurred some years after excellent histological reversal of active lupus glomerulonephritis at a time when the renal biopsy was normal and there was no proteinuria or hypertension. Such patients usually have successful pregnancies without complications. We often maintain our lupus nephritis patients on a small dose of prednisolone, 7.5–10 mg daily, indefinitely if withdrawal of treatment is associated

Table 6.7.1–6   Comparison of maternal outcome of pregnancies in lupus anticoagulant (LAC) positive and negative mothers (from Packham et al 1992, with permission)

Maternal outcome	LAC +ve (n = 21)		LAC –ve (n = 43)	
	No.	%	No.	%
Impaired renal function				
Irreversible	0	–	1	2
Reversible	7	33	4	9
Total	7	33	5	12
Hypertension				
Irreversible	2	10	7	16
Reversible	4	19	11	26
Exacerbation	3	14	1	2
Total	9	43	19	44
Early	8	38	10	23
Severe	3	14	5	12
Increased protenuria				
Irreversible	0	–	3	7
Reversible	9	43	19	44
Total	9	43	22	51

with an increase in the urinary erythrocyte count or in proteinuria.

Steroids were being administered during pregnancy in 67% of patients.

Depending on the severity of the renal lesion, we also frequently treat patients with aspirin and/or dipyridamole for their antithrombotic effects.

Table 6.7.1–7   Treatment of lupus glomerulonephritis during pregnancy

	No.	%
Prednisolone	43	67
Heparin	16	25
Aspirin	12	19
Dipyridamole	10	16
Azathioprine	8	13
Plasma exchange	5	8
Gammaglobulin (in patients LAC +ve)	4	6
Eicosapentaenoic acid	3	5

We have demonstrated benefit in a controlled trial in patients with renal disease using a combination of heparin and dipyridamole. In patients with more severe glomerular lesions such as crescents, we have used this combination of heparin and dipyridamole or plasma exchange.

Table 6.7.1–7 shows the treatment used during pregnancy in the patients with lupus glomerulonephritis.

In lupus glomerulonephritis, as in other forms of glomerulonephritis, we have observed the development of crescents on renal biopsy during pregnancy. In this group of patients with lupus glomerulonephritis 10 biopsies were carried out during pregnancy and 3 (30%) showed crescents.

Our results in this series of 64 pregnancies in 41 women with biopsy proven lupus glomerulonephritis compare favourably with other series in terms of fetal outcome. In the only other large series from one institution (Bobrie et al 1987) fetal loss in women with lupus nephritis (excluding those where pregnancies preceded the clinical onset of lupus) was 28 of 67 fetuses (42%). Cameron & Hicks (1984) in their review recorded a fetal loss of 26%. Hayslett & Lynn (1980) in a review of results in a mail survey of nephrologists recorded an overall fetal loss of 38%. Mintz & Rodriquez-Alvarez (1989) found no difference in fetal loss in 44 pregnancies in women with systemic lupus erythematosus without nephritis and 58 pregnancies in women with nephritis (see Table 6.7.1–8).

In view of the striking influence of the presence of circulating lupus anticoagulant on fetal outcome it would be of interest to know the lupus anticoagulant status of the patients in Table 6.7.1–8.

The maternal outcome in our series is excellent with neither end stage renal failure nor death occurring in any patient.

Cameron & Hicks (1984) reported a maternal death rate of 3.4% in 345 pregnancies in 218 women. In Bobrie et al's (1987) large study, 6 of 53 pregnancies were associated with severe deterioration in renal function and 4 rapidly developed end stage renal failure. Of 19 women reported by Imbasciati et al (1984) 4 developed acute renal failure in the postpartum period and 2 of these died. We have reported postpartum renal failure and features of a thrombotic microangiopathy in women with a circulating lupus anticoagulant, only 2 of whom had lupus nephritis (Kincaid-Smith et al 1988). Possibly this mechanism was responsible for postpartum renal failure in some of the acute renal failure cases

Table 6.7.1–8   Outcome of pregnancy (from Mintz & Rodriquez-Alvarez 1989, with permission)

	Abortions		Prematurity		Intrauterine malnutrition		Perinatal mortality	
	No	%	No.	%	No.	%	No.	%
Without nephropathy (44 pregnancies)	5 (3 active SLE and infections)	11.3	20	45	9	20	2	4.5
With nephropathy (58 pregnancies)	12 (4 active SLE, 4 infections, 1 fibroma, 2 hypertension)	20.6	25	43	11	19	3	5.1

SLE, systemic lupus erythematosus.

reported by Bobrie et al (1987) and Imbasciati et al (1984).

These frequent records of maternal deaths and end stage renal failure together with Bear's (1976) recorded mortality in 3 of 6 patients warrant a cautious attitude in lupus nephritis.

Perhaps the reason why we recorded no maternal mortality or end stage renal disease is because the majority of our pregnancies (46/64) took place in patients in whom we had previously documented lupus nephritis. Our policy in such patients would be to treat the renal lesion aggressively to achieve reversal of the histological abnormalities. We are usually able to achieve this and we would not advise pregnancy until the renal biopsy was inactive; in many cases in this series the renal biopsy would have been normal or almost normal at the commencement of pregnancy. Lupus nephritis is one of the most responsive forms of glomerulonephritis in our experience (Leaker et al 1987). Such patients would also usually have no proteinuria and an inactive urinary sediment with a low urinary erythrocyte count. Perhaps we were lucky not to encounter serious problems in the 18 pregnancies in which the patient presented during pregnancy. Active treatment detailed in Table 6.7.1–7, including plasma exchange in some with more severe renal lesions, may have averted deterioration in renal function in some patients. One patient who presented with severe postpartum renal failure was stabilized on plasma exchange and still had stable renal function 16 years later.

The question as to whether pregnancy causes an exacerbation of activity in systemic lupus erythematosus seems to have been answered by three recent controlled studies, none of which suggest that pregnancy causes an exacerbation of systemic lupus erythematosus (Meehan & Dorsey 1987, Lockshin et al 1984, Mintz & Rodriguez-Alvarez 1989).

The occurrence of neonatal systemic lupus transmitted by transfer of antinuclear antibodies from mother to fetus should be borne in mind. Cardiac and haematological abnormalities are those most frequently observed in the fetus. Heart block due to antinuclear antibodies in the conducting system of the fetus is the most serious complication.

The syndrome is self limiting as it is due to passive transfer of antibodies. It is rarely encountered if the mother is on adequate treatment for her systemic lupus.

REFERENCES

Bear R 1976 Pregnancy and lupus nephritis — a detailed report of six cases with a review of the literature. Obstetrics and Gynecology 47: 715–718

Bear R A 1978 Pregnancy in patients with chronic renal disease. Canadian Medical Association Journal 118: 663–669

Bobrie G, Liote F, Houillier P et al 1987 Pregnancy in lupus nephritis and related disorders. American Journal of Kidney Diseases 9: 339–343

Cameron J S, Hicks J 1984 Pregnancy in patients with pre-existing glomerular disease. Contributions to Nephrology 37: 149–156

Hayslett J P, Lynn R I 1980 Effect of pregnancy in patients with lupus nephropathy. Kidney International 18: 207–220

Imbasciati E, Surian M, Bottino S et al 1984 Lupus nephropathy and pregnancy. Nephron 36: 46–51

Kincaid-Smith P 1967 The clinical value of renal biopsy. In: G E Schreiner (ed) 3rd International Congress of Nephrology, 1966. Morphology, immunology, urology. Karger, Basel, vol 2: p 178–197

Kincaid-Smith P, Fairley K F, Kloss M 1988 Lupus anticoagulant associated with renal thrombotic microangiopathy and pregnancy-related renal failure. Quarterly Journal of Medicine 258: 795–815

Leaker B, Fairley K F, Dowling J et al 1987 Lupus nephritis: clinical and pathological correlation. Quarterly Journal of Medicine 238: 163–179

Lockshin M D, Reinitz E, Druzin M L, et al 1984 Lupus pregnancy. American Journal of Medicine 77: 893–898

Meehan R T, Dorsey J K 1987 Pregnancy among patients with systemic lupus erythematosus receiving immunosuppressive therapy. Journal of Rheumatology 14: 252–258

Mintz G, Rodriques-Alvarez E 1989 Systemic lupus erythematosus. Rheumatic Diseases Clinics of North America 15: 255–274

Packham D K, Lam S S, Nicholls K et al 1992 Lupus nephritis and pregnancy. Quarterly Journal of Medicine 83: 315–324

6.7.2 Lupus anticoagulant and anti-phospholipid antibodies (anticardiolipin antibodies)

Whether it is associated with other features of systemic lupus erythematosus and lupus glomerulonephritis or not, the presence of a circulating lupus anticoagulant or the presence in the serum of antiphospholipid or anticardiolipin antibodies may have very serious implications for the outcome of pregnancy.

The major interest in the presence of a lupus anticoagulant in the past has been its association with thrombotic lesions (Bowie et al 1963, Mueh et al 1980, Boey et al 1983, Harris et al 1983, Elias et al 1984). More recently interest has centred on the very high incidence of fetal loss in pregnant women with a circulating lupus anticoagulant or antiphospholipid antibodies (Nilsson et al 1975, Firkin et al 1980, Carreras et al 1981, Garlund 1984, Fraga et al 1984, Feinstein 1985, Branch et al 1985, Lubbe & Liggins 1985, Lockshin et al 1987, Ordi et al 1989, Gatenby et al 1989, Kincaid-Smith et al 1988).

Patients with the circulating coagulation inhibitor which has been termed 'lupus anticoagulant' show lesions in the microvasculature of the kidney (Kincaid-Smith et al 1988) and the placenta (De Wolf et al 1982) which resemble those seen in preeclampsia although they are more severe and extensive. In particular, the vascular lesions in the placenta described by De Wolf (1982) are very similar to the specific lesions in placental vessels described in preeclampsia (Robertson et al 1976). Fetal loss is likely to be due to the placental vessel lesions and resultant extensive placental infarction.

In a series of 12 women with a lupus anticoagulant in whom only 2 of 23 pregnancies were successful, we found acute fibrin thrombi in glomeruli and renal arteries and arterioles in all 7 renal biopsies taken during or soon after pregnancy (Kincaid-Smith et al 1988). The acute lesions associated with fibrin thrombi in arteries, arterioles and glomeruli on light microscopy showed ultrastructural changes characteristic of the haemolytic uraemic syndrome or postpartum renal failure (Fig. 6.3.3–3). Vascular lesions were demonstrated on biopsy as early as 6 weeks after the commencement of pregnancy, and chronic lesions persisted in vessels for as long as 10 years after the biopsy demonstration of the acute lesions. These late lesions consisted of recanalized thrombi and severe narrowing of the lumen by cellular and fibroelastic intimal thickening (Fig. 6.7.2–1). Characteristic double contours were seen persisting in glomeruli for months after the acute phase (Fig. 6.3.3–4).

Impaired renal function was documented in this series of patients both in the acute phase and subsequently; 4 patients had severely impaired renal function and 2 showed moderate impairment of renal function. Treatment by plasma

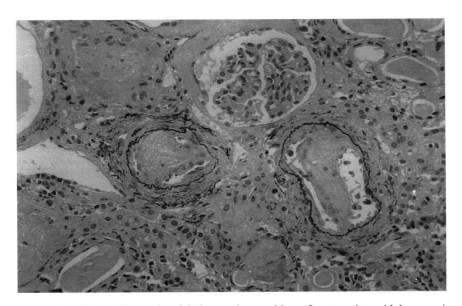

Fig. 6.7.2–1 Recanalization of thrombi in two interlobular arteries on a biopsy from a patient with lupus anticoagulant who developed acute vascular lesions during pregnancy.

exchange in the early postpartum period when the acute fibrinoid lesions were present was associated with rapid improvement in renal function.

One of our patients died from massive haemorrhage following an exploration laparotomy. Severe haemorrhagic complications have been documented in other patients with a lupus anticoagulant (Manoharan & Gottliel 1984, Ordi et al 1984).

Prostacyclin deficiency has been suggested as one mechanism leading to thrombosis (Carreras et al 1981). Other mechanisms such as an inhibitor of the protein C anticoagulant pathway (Amer et al 1990) have been proposed as an explanation for thrombotic episodes.

Treatment with high dose steroids has achieved a far greater percentage of successful pregnancies in women with a lupus anticoagulant (Lubbe et al 1983). In 2 of our patients treated with steroids there was a suggestion that prolonging the pregnancy by the use of steroids may have aggravated the vascular lesions (Kincaid-Smith et al 1988).

A far simpler treatment with low dose aspirin (75–150 mg/day) reduced the fetal loss from 88% to 55% in patients with systemic lupus erythematosus and phospholipid antibodies. In the same study, in patients with phospholipid antibodies but no manifestation of systemic lupus, the fetal loss improved from 79% to 25% following aspirin treatment (Gatenby et al 1989). We can confirm these results using aspirin and using a combination of aspirin and dipyridamole. In more serious cases with renal vascular lesions we have achieved good results using steroids, heparin and dipyridamole or plasma exchange.

REFERENCES

Amer L, Kisiel W, Searles R P et al 1990 Impairment of the protein C anticoagulant pathway in a patient with systemic lupus erythematosus, anticardiolipin antibodies and thrombosis. Thrombosis Research 57: 247–258

Boey M L, Colaco C B, Gharavi A E et al 1983 Thrombosis in systemic lupus erythematosus: striking association with the presence of circulating lupus 'anticoagulant'. British Medical Journal 287: 1021–1023

Bowie E J, Thompson J H Jr, Pascuzzie C A et al 1963 Thrombosis in systemic lupus erythematosus despite circulating anticoagulants. Journal of Laboratory and Clinical Medicine 62: 416–430

Branch D W, Scott J P, Kochenour N K et al 1985 Obstetric complications associated with lupus anticoagulant. New England Journal of Medicine 313: 1322–1326

Carreras L O, Vermylen J, Spitz B et al 1981 Lupus anticoagulant and inhibition of prostacyclin formation in patients with repeated abortion, intrauterine growth retardation and intrauterine death. British Journal of Obstetrics and Gynaecology 88: 890–894

De Wolf F, Carreras L O, Moerman P et al 1982 Decidual vasculopathy and extensive placental infarction in a patient with repeated thromboembolic accidents, recurrent foetal loss and a lupus anticoagulant. American Journal of Obstetrics and Gynecology 142: 829–834

Elias M, Eldor A 1984 Thromboembolism in patients with the 'lupus' type circulating anticoagulant. Archives of Internal Medicine 144: 510–515

Feinstein D I 1985 Thrombosis and fetal loss. New England Journal of Medicine 313: 1348–1350

Firkin B G, Howard M A, Radford N 1980 Possible relationship between lupus anticoagulant and recurrent abortion in young women. Lancet 2: 366

Fraga A, Mintz G, Orozco J et al 1984 Sterility and fertility rates, foetal wastage and maternal morbidity in systemic lupus erythematosus. Journal of Rheumatology 1: 293–298

Garlund B 1984 The lupus inhibitor in thromboembolic disease and intrauterine death in the absence of systemic lupus. Acta Medica Scandinavica 215: 293–298

Gatenby P A, Cameron K, Shearman R P 1989 Pregnancy loss with phospholipid antibodies: Improved outcome with aspirin containing treatment. Australian and New Zealand Journal of Obstetrics and Gynaecology 29: 294–298

Harris E N, Gharavie A E, Boey M L et al 1983 Anticardiolipin antibodies: detection by radio-immunoassay and association with thrombosis in systemic lupus erythematosus. Lancet 2: 1211–1214

Kincaid-Smith P, Fairley K F, Kloss M 1988 Lupus anticoagulant associated with renal thrombotic microangiopathy and pregnancy related renal failure. Quarterly Journal of Medicine 258: 795–815

Lockshin M D, Qamar T, Druzin M L et al 1987 Antibody to cardiolipin, lupus anticoagulant, and fetal death. Journal of Rheumatology 14: 259–262

Lubbe W F, Liggins G C 1985 Anticoagulant and pregnancy. American Journal of Obstetrics and Gynecology 153: 422–327

Lubbe W F, Butler W S, Palmer S J et al 1983 Fetal survival after prednisone suppression of maternal lupus-anticoagulant. Lancet 1: 1361–1363

Manoharan A, Gottlieb P 1984 Bleeding in patients with lupus anticoagulant. Lancet 2: 171

Mueh J R, Herbst K D, Rapaport S I 1980 Thrombosis in patients with the lupus 'anticoagulant'. Annals of Internal Medicine 92: 156–159

Nilsson I M, Astedt B, Hedner U et al 1975 Intrauterine death and circulating anticoagulant ('Antithromboplastin'). Acta Medica Scandinavica 197: 153–159

Ordi J, Vilardel M, Oristrell J et al 1984 Bleeding in patients with lupus anticoagulant. Lancet 2: 868–869

Ordi J, Barquinero J, Vilardell M et al 1989 Fetal loss treatment in patients with antiphospholipid antibodies. Annals of the Rheumatic Diseases 48: 798–802

Robertson W B, Brosens I, Dixon G 1976 Maternal uterine vascular lesions in the hypertensive complications of pregnancy. In: M D Lindheimer, A I Katz, F E Zuspan (eds) Hypertension in pregnancy. Wiley, New York, p 115

6.7.3   Pregnancy in women with glomerulonephritis and vascular lesions in the kidney associated with systemic disease

Henoch–Schönlein syndrome, Goodpasture's syndrome, polyarteritis nodosa and scleroderma

In a number of systemic diseases, glomerular and vascular lesions are present in the kidney. Most important among these diseases in the context of pregnancy is systemic lupus erythematosus, because this is typically a disease of young women (this disease is dealt with in 6.7.1 and 6.7.2).

Henoch–Schönlein syndrome may have associated glomerulonephritis. It is a rare condition in adults — we have little experience of this disorder in pregnancy and could find no published series of cases. The glomerular lesions in this syndrome are very similar to those in mesangial IgA glomerulonephritis, although the lesions are more frequently crescentic and the prognosis is generally regarded as poor (Anonymous 1971).

Goodpasture's syndrome is another rare disorder which is almost always fatal if untreated. Very few data are available on the outcome in pregnancy in recovered cases. Goodpasture's syndrome usually presents with a combination of pulmonary haemorrhage and fulminating glomerulonephritis which progresses rapidly to end stage renal failure. Recovery was rarely recorded prior to the advent of plasma exchange, but up to 40% of patients may now have a good long term recovery of renal function (Walker et al 1984).

Among our patients, 3 young women who recovered following plasma exchange and now have normal renal function have had successful pregnancies with only minor maternal complications in spite of destruction of over 80% of glomeruli by crescents in 2 of these 3 women during the acute stage of this disease.

Polyarteritis nodosa is another rare condition and only a handful of reports of pregnancy in women with this condition are available. Siegler & Spain (1965) reported a case and reviewed the literature in 1965. Of 5 young women aged 23–39 recorded in this review all died soon after pregnancy although the pregnancy was successful in achieving a live infant in 4 cases.

Steroid therapy is often dramatically effective in polyarteritis nodosa and in subsequent reports 6 patients who had been treated with steroids and were in remission at the onset of pregnancy all survived. There were 2 therapeutic abortions and 1 late fetal death, but 3 pregnancies were successful (Owen & Hauth 1989).

In this later report (Owen & Hauth 1989) a further 2 cases were reviewed in which the disease had presented during pregnancy or in the puerperium as it did in the 5 cases reviewed by Siegler & Spain (1965). These additional 2 patients who presented with acute manifestations during pregnancy, also died in the postpartum period as did the 5 women reported by Siegler & Spain (1965).

Thus 7 of 12 women with polyarteritis nodosa had a successful pregnancy but died in the puerperium. This suggests that an exacerbation of this disease may occur in late pregnancy or in the early postpartum period. We have seen an additional patient with polyarteritis nodosa, who presented with severe hypertension in pregnancy and developed vascular complications and died soon after delivery. The pathology in this case suggested a recent acute exacerbation of arteritic lesions. Fresh fibrinoid necrosis was also illustrated at autopsy in 1 case by Siegler & Spain (1965).

Scleroderma is another condition in which pregnancy may precipitate a crisis. Alteri & Cameron (1988) recently reviewed reports of women with scleroderma who developed a renal crisis in relation to pregnancy. In this report all the mothers died days to months after the pregnancy except the patient reported by Alteri & Cameron (1988) who was treated with heparin and dipyridamole, captopril and haemodialysis. Late recovery of renal function in this patient permitted withdrawal of dialysis.

The scleroderma crisis, accompanied by malignant hypertension with or without a frank thrombotic microangiopathy, developed in the third trimester or in the early postpartum period in all reported cases (Table 6.7.3–1).

Although recovery of renal function following scleroderma crisis has been reported in other patients treated with converting enzyme inhibitors (Lopez-Ovejero et al 1979), Alteri & Cameron's case is the only recorded recovery where the crisis arose in pregnancy or the early postpartum period. A successful pregnancy has,

Table 6.7.3–1   Scleroderma crisis with renal failure in relation to pregnancy (from Altieri & Cameron 1988, with permission)

Study	Age	Race	Timing of crisis	BP (max.)	MAHA	Anticoagulation	Duration of renal failure	Treatment	Outcome
Fear 1968	26	C	Third trimester	240/130	No	No	21 days until death	Pred:BP	Death
Sood & Kohler 1970	25	C	Third trimester	200/126	No	No	9 days until death	Pred: BP	Death
Karlen & Cook 1974	26	C	Third trimester	200/125	No	No	7 days until death	Pred: BP	Death
Ehrenfeld et al 1977	20	?	3 weeks pp	260/160	No	No	17 months until death	Pred: BP	Death
Smith & Pinals 1982	25	C	1 day pp	170/140	No	No	4 months until death	Pred: BP	Triple amputation: death
Present case	34	C	Third trimester	210/110	Yes	Yes	14 months	ACE	Recovered some function

C, Caucasian; PP, postpartum; MAHA, microangiopathic haemolytic anaemia; Pred, prednis(ol)one; BP, conventional hypotensive; ACE, angiotensin converting enzyme inhibitor.

Table 6.7.3–2   Pregnancy outcome in progressive systemic sclerosis (from Scarpinato & Mackenzie 1985, with permission)

Mother and child normal			Fetal death (Maternal condition stable)			Maternal death (usually also fetal loss)		
No. of patients	Study	Year	No. of patients	Study	Year	No. of patients	Study	Year
1	Anselmino & Hoffmann	1932	1	Eno	1937	1	Etterich & Mall	1964
1	Eno	1937	1	Leinwand et al	1954	1	Casten & Boucek	1958
1	Guttmacher	1943	1	Hayes et al	1962	1	Slate & Graham	1967
1	Leinwand et al	1954	1	Spellacy	1964	1	Donaldson	1967
1	Tischler et al	1957	1	Johnson et al	1964	1	Fear	1968
1	Hoffman & Diamond	1961	2	Slate & Graham	1967	1	Sood & Kohler	1970
1	Winkleman	1962	1	Donaldson	1967	1	Karlen & Cook	1974
36	Johnson et al	1964	1	Watson et al	1981	1	Ehrenfeld et al	1977
1	Gunther & Harer	1964	1	Thompson & Conklin	1983	1	Garcez et al*	1979
3	Slate & Graham	1967				1	Palma et al*	1981
3	Donaldson	1967				1	Smith & Pinals	1982
1	Knupp & O'Leary	1971				1	Mor-Yosef et al	1984
2	Spiera	1981						
1	Sivanesaratnam & Chong	1982						
1	Goplerud	1983						
1	Mor-Yosef et al	1984						
3	Ballou et al	1984						
1	Scarpinato & Mackenzie	1985						

* No fetal death.
Fetal wastage = fetal death + (maternal death – no fetal death)/total.

however, been reported in a woman in whom an earlier course of treatment with converting enzyme inhibitors had reversed a hypertensive crisis (Spiera et al 1989).

The overall results of pregnancy in patients with scleroderma are less dramatic than those in which a crisis develops but there is still a serious maternal mortality rate and high fetal loss. Scarpinato &

Mackenzie (1985) found 82 published reports, the results of which are summarized in Table 6.7.3–2. 15% of cases resulted in maternal death usually as a result of accelerated hypertension and post-partum renal failure. Fetal loss was recorded as 23%, excluding spontaneous abortions.

REFERENCES

Altieri P, Cameron J S 1988 Scleroderma renal crisis in a pregnant woman with late partial recovery of renal function. Nephrology, Dialysis, Transplantation 3: 677–680

Anonymous 1971 Henoch–Schönlein purpura and the kidneys. British Medical Journal 2: 352

Anselmino K J, Hoffmann F 1932 Uber Sklerodermi und Schwangerschaft. Zeitschrift fuer Geburtshilfe und Gynaekologie 103: 60–66

Ballou S P, Morley J J, Kuchner I 1984 Pregnancy and systemic sclerosis. Arthritis and Rheumatism 27: 295–298

Casten G G, Boucek R J 1958 Use of relaxin in the treatment of systemic scleroderma. Journal of the American Medical Association 166: 319–329

Donaldson L B in Slate & Graham 1967

Ehrenfeld M, Licht A, Stessman J et al 1977 Postpartum renal failure due to progressive systemic sclerosis treated with chronic haemodialysis. Nephron 18: 175–181

Eno E 1937 Pregnancy in a patient suffering with scleroderma. American Journal of Obstetrics and Gynecology 33: 514–515

Etterich M, Mall M 1964 Scleroderma and pregnancy: report of a case. Obstetrics and Gynecology 23: 297–300

Fear R E 1968 Eclampsia superimposed on renal scleroderma: a rare cause of maternal and fetal mortality. Obstetrics and Gynecology 31: 69–74

Garcez D de M, Costa C, Prompt C A 1979 Gestation and rapidly progressive form of scleroderma. Revista da Associacao Medica Brasileira 25: 445–446

Goplerud C P. 1983 Scleroderma. Clinical Obstetrics and Gynecology 26: 587–591

Gunther R E, Harer Jr W B 1964 Systemic scleroderma in pregnancy: report of a case. Obstetrics and Gynecology 24: 98–100

Guttmacher A F 1943 A case of severe scleroderma with successful delivery. Urologic and Cutaneous Review 47: 107–108

Hayes G W, Walsh C R, D'Alessandro E E 1962 Scleroderma in pregnancy: report of a case. Obstetrics and Gynecology 19: 273–274

Hoffman J B, Diamond B 1961 Scleroderma treated with steroids through pregnancy, cesarean section and puerperium. Postgraduate Medicine 30: 498–501

Johnson T R, Banner E A, Winkelmann R K 1964 Scleroderma and pregnancy. Obstetrics and Gynecology 23: 467–469

Karlen J R, Cook W A 1974 Renal scleroderma and pregnancy. Obstetrics and Gynecology 44: 349–354

Knupp M Z, O'Leary J A 1971 Pregnancy and scleroderma: systemic sclerosis. Journal of the Florida Medical Association 58: 28–30

Leinwand I, Duryee A W, Richter M N 1954 Scleroderma (based on a study of over 150 cases). Annals of Internal Medicine 41: 1003–1041

Lopez-Ovejero J A, Saal S D, D'Angelo W A et al 1979 Reversal of vascular and renal crisis by oral angiotensin-converting-enzyme blockade. New England Journal of Medicine 300: 1417–1419

Mor-Yosef S, Navot D, Rabinowitz R et al 1984 Collagen diseases in pregnancy. Obstetric and Gynecological Survey 39: 67–84

Owen J, Hauth J C, 1989 Polyarteritis nodosa in pregnancy: a case report and brief literature review. American Journal of Obstetrics and Gynecology 160: 606–607

Palma A, Sanchez-Palencia A, Armas J R et al 1981 Progressive systemic sclerosis and nephrotic syndrome: an unusual association resulting in postpartum acute renal failure. Archives of Internal Medicine 141: 521–522

Scarpinato L, MacKenzie A H 1985 Pregnancy and progressive systemic sclerosis: case report and review of the literature. Cleveland Clinic Journal of Medicine 52: 207–211

Siegler A M, Spain D M 1965 Polyarteritis nodosa and pregnancy. Clinical Obstetrics and Gynecology 8: 322–333

Sivanesaratnam V, Chong H L 1982 Scleroderma and pregnancy. Australian and New Zealand Journal of Obstetrics and Gynaecology 22: 123–124

Slate W G, Graham A R 1967 Scleroderma and pregnancy. American Journal of Obstetrics and Gynecology 101: 335–341

Smith C A, Pinals R S 1982 Progressive systemic sclerosis and postpartum renal failure complicated by peripheral gangrene. Journal of Rheumatology 9: 455–458

Sood S V, Kohler H G 1970 Maternal death from systemic sclerosis (report of a case of renal scleroderma masquerading as pre-eclamptic toxaemia). Journal of Obstetrics and Gynaecology of the British Commonwealth 77: 1109–1112

Spellacy W N 1964 Scleroderma and pregnancy: report of a case. Obstetrics and Gynaecology 23: 297–300

Spiera H 1981 The clinical picture of connective tissue diseases in pregnancy. Progress Clinical and Biological Research 70: 303–307

Spiera H, Krakoff L, Fishbane-Mayer J 1989 Successful pregnancy after scleroderma hypertensive renal crisis. Journal of Rheumatology 16: 1597–1598

Thompson J, Conklin K A, 1983 Anaesthetic management of a pregnant patient with scleroderma. Anesthesiology 59: 69–71

Tischler S, Zarowitz H, Daichman I 1957 Scleroderma and pregnancy. Obstetrics and Gynecology 10: 457–459

Walker R G, Scheinkestel C, Becker G J et al 1984 Clinical and morphological aspects of the management of crescentic anti-glomerular basement membrane antibody (anti-GBM) nephritis/Goodpasture's syndrome. Quarterly Journal of Medicine 34: 96–97

Watson M A, Radford N J, McGrath B P et al 1981 Captopril-induced agranulocytosis in systemic sclerosis. Australian and New Zealand Journal of Medicine 11: 79–81

Winkleman E 1962 Pregnancy in advanced systemic scleroderma. Journal of the American Medical Association 17: 557–561

6.8   RENAL ARTERY STENOSIS AND LESIONS IN THE RENAL MICROVASCULATURE IN RELATION TO PREGNANCY AND PREECLAMPSIA

6.8.1   Renal artery stenosis

There have been relatively few reports of pregnancy in women with renal artery stenosis. Although the multicentre study in the United States suggested that renal artery stenosis is a relatively common cause of hypertension (Simon et al 1972), the majority of cases are due to atheroma. Atheromatous renal artery stenosis is very rare in women under 50 years of age and cases of renal artery stenosis in pregnancy belong to the pathological categories grouped under the title 'fibromuscular hyperplasia'.

Easterling et al (1991) recently reported 2 further cases of renal artery stenosis who presented during pregnancy, and reviewed previous reports (Wylie & Wellington 1960, Hunt et al 1962, Koskela & Kaski 1971, Hotchkiss et al 1971, Roach 1973, McCarron et al 1982, Sellars et al 1985). 68% of patients (including the 2 reported by Easterling (1991) had hypertension in the first trimester — not a surprising observation because the lesion clearly preceded pregnancy. Hypertension is often severe and led to termination of pregnancy in 3 cases. In 9 of 16 reported pregnancies the diastolic blood pressure was 110 mmHg or higher.

The fetal outlook is poor. Among 11 pregnancies for which data are available, 3 were terminated because of severe hypertension and there was 1 spontaneous abortion and 2 stillbirths; 2 required caesarean section for fetal distress and 2 of 3 patients who had uncomplicated successful deliveries had percutaneous transluminal dilatation of the renal artery performed during pregnancy.

One of the 2 patients reported by Easterling et al (1991) had correction of the renal artery lesion by transluminal angioplasty at 20 weeks' gestation. Before this procedure, this patient had a very high vascular resistance which fell significantly after the angioplasty. The blood pressure fell to levels of 150–134 mmHg systolic and 70–85 mmHg diastolic after dilatation of the renal artery lesion, whereas the blood pressure at presentation at 8 weeks' gestation had been 180/120 mmHg; so that substantial clinical benefit was achieved by the procedure.

Our own experience of renal artery stenosis in pregnancy is limited to 2 cases, both of which had very severe hypertension.

6.8.2   Lesions in the renal microvasculature in relation to pregnancy and preeclampsia

In patients with underlying renal disease and in patients with preeclampsia, vascular lesions may be seen in biopsies taken during pregnancy. The acute features of these vascular lesions, which may contain fibrin or fibrinoid material, indicate that they have developed during pregnancy (Kincaid-Smith 1975a). They may be seen in patients with a normal blood pressure, and the fact that they appear during pregnancy can be documented in serial biopsies (Kincaid-Smith 1973).

Burden et al (1979) demonstrated vascular lesions angiographically after complicated pregnancies, and their studies, like ours, suggest that it is unlikely that hypertension played any significant role in the appearance of these vascular lesions during pregnancy.

Vascular lesions which appear to be independent of hypertension are also seen in a variety of types of glomerulonephritis in non- pregnant patients (Kincaid-Smith et al 1973, Kincaid-Smith 1975a).

We believe that intravascular coagulation in the kidney plays a part in the formation of these vascular lesions (Kincaid-Smith 1975b).

Apart from Burden et al's (1979) angiographic studies, Abe et al's biopsy study (1985) and Gaber & Spargo's (1987) observations of vascular lesions in association with focal glomerulosclerosis and Abe's report, there has been little reference to the occurrence of these vascular lesions in association with pregnancy.

We recently described a series of biopsies in patients with a circulating lupus anticoagulant (Kincaid-Smith et al 1988). Biopsies taken during pregnancy or in the early postpartum period showed fibrin deposited in arteries and arterioles in the kidney, 25 follow up biopsies in these patients showed persisting fibroelastic and fibrocellular intimal thickening in vessels in the kidney for periods of up to 10 years. These lesions are associated with a coagulation abnormality which is known to produce thrombotic lesions, and the demonstration of thrombi in vessels which evolve in serial biopsies into recanalized and then permanent fibrocellular or fibroelastic lesions strengthens our belief that a similar but less severe process is responsible for the vascular lesions which develop in preeclampsia. Preeclampsia is also a condition in which intravascular coagulation is well documented as it is in association with a circulating lupus anticoagulant.

Both in patients who have had prior pre-eclampsia and in those with renal disease, we have been able to correctly predict the likely recurrence of preeclampsia or superimposed pre-eclampsia on the basis of the extent and severity of these vascular lesions seen on renal biopsy.

In our large series of patients with glomerulo-nephritis, we have found that the presence and severity of vascular lesions influences the likelihood of fetal loss (Fig. 6.8.2–1).

Maternal outcome in terms of impaired renal function, hypertension and increased proteinuria showed a higher percentage of abnormalities in women whose biopsies showed severe vessel lesions, but these did not reach statistical significance (Packham et al 1989).

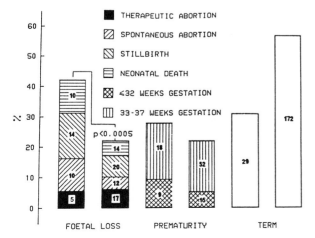

Fig. 6.8.2–1 Fetal outcome of pregnancies in women with severe vessel lesions (left-hand column) and mild to moderate lesions (right-hand column).

REFERENCES

Abe S, Amagasaki Y, Konishi K et al 1985 The influence of antecedent renal disease on pregnancy. American Journal of Obstetrics and Gynecology 153: 508–514

Burden R P, Boyd W N, Aber G M 1979 Structural and functional changes in the renal circulation after complicated pregnancy. Nephron 24: 183–1192

Easterling T R, Goldman M L, Strandness D E et al 1991 Renal vascular hypertension during pregnancy. Obstetrics and Gynecology 78: 921–925

Gaber L W, Spargo B 1987 Pregnancy-induced nephropathy: the significance of focal segmental glomerulosclerosis. American Journal of Kidney Diseases 9: 317–323

Hotchkiss R L, Nettles J B, Wells D E 1971 Renovascular hypertension in pregnancy. Southern Medical Journal 64: 1256–1258

Hunt J C, Harrison Jr E G, Kincaid O W, 1962 Idiopathic fibrous and fibromuscular stenoses of the renal arteries associated with hypertension. Proceedings of the Mayo Clinic 37: 181–216

Kincaid-Smith P 1973 The similarity of lesions and underlying mechanism in preeclamptic toxaemia and post-partum renal failure. Studies in the acute stage and during follow-up. In: P Kincaid-Smith, T H Mathew, E L Becker (eds) Glomerulonephritis. Wiley, New York, p 1013–1025

Kincaid-Smith P 1975a The kidney — a clinicopathological study. Blackwell Scientific, Oxford, p 193, 227

Kincaid-Smith P 1975b Participation of intravascular coagulation in the pathogenesis of glomerular and vascular lesions. Kidney International 7: 242–253

Kincaid-Smith P, Mathew T H, Becker E L (eds) 1973 Glomerulonephritis. Wiley, New York, p 157

Kincaid-Smith P, Fairley K F, Kloss M 1988 Lupus anticoagulant associated with renal thrombotic microangiopathy and pregnancy related renal failure. Quarterly Journal of Medicine 69: 795–815

Koskela O, Kaski P 1971 Renal angiography in the follow-up examination of toxaemia of late pregnancy. Acta Obstetricia et Gynecologica Scandinavica 50: 41–43

McCarron D A, Keller F S, Lundquist G et al 1982 Transluminal angioplasty for renovascular hypertension complicated by pregnancy. Archives of Internal Medicine 142: 1737–1738

Packham D K, North R A, Fairley K F et al 1989 Primary glomerulonephritis and pregnancy. Quarterly Journal of Medicine 71: 537–553

Roach C J 1973 Renovascular hypertension in pregnancy. Obstetrics and Gynecology 42: 856–860

Sellars L, Siamopoulos K, Wilkinson R 1985 Prognosis for pregnancy after correction of renovascular hypertension. Nephron 39: 280–281

Simon N, Franklin S S, Bleifer K H et al 1972 Clinical characteristics of renovascular hypertension. Journal of the American Medical Association 220: 1209–1218

Wylie E J, Wellington J S 1960 Hypertension caused by fibromuscular hyperplasia of the renal arteries. American Journal of Surgery 100: 183–193

6.9 DIABETIC RENAL DISEASE AND PREGNANCY

In early studies Simms & Krantz (1958) found no evidence of deterioration in renal function during pregnancy in women with diabetes. White (1965) and Oppe et al (1957), on the other hand, considered that pregnancy aggravated the course of patients with diabetic nephropathy.

Following Kitzmiller's important papers of a decade ago (Kitzmiller et al 1978, 1981), Hayslett's group (Reece et al 1988, Hayslett & Reece 1987a, b) have been the major recent contributors on the topic of pregnancy and diabetic nephropathy: however, Combs & Kitzmiller (1991) recently reviewed this topic.

Kitzmiller's study in 1978 of pregnancy outcome in 147 women with diabetes attending the Joslin Clinic in Boston was a major contribution on pregnancy and perinatal outcome in diabetes but made little mention of diabetic nephropathy. Pedersen & Pedersen (1965) had reported a high prevalence of urinary tract infection (16%) and acute pyelonephritis (6%) in diabetic pregnant women, but Kitzmiller encountered pyelonephritis in only 1% of his large series.

Other maternal complications reported by Kitzmiller et al are shown in Table 6.9–1, which indicates a surprisingly low incidence of pre-eclampsia (5%) and hypertension.

Kitzmiller's second study (1981) examined the influence of diabetic nephropathy on perinatal outcome and on hypertension and renal function in 35 women with diabetic nephropathy attending the Joslin clinic. Spontaneous or elective abortion occurred in 25% of cases and 71% of deliveries occurred before 37 weeks; neonatal deaths occurred in 11% of cases. The birth weight was dependent on the maternal blood pressure and creatinine clearance (Fig. 6.9–1).

Maternal proteinuria increased to over 3 g/24 h in 69% of pregnancies and this persisted after pregnancy at the same level in 26%. Proteinuria was above 6 g/24 h in 57% of cases and this very high level persisted after pregnancy in 17%.

Decreased renal function defined as a serum creatinine above 1.5 mg/100 ml was noted during pregnancy in 30% of cases and this degree of functional impairment was present at follow up in an even higher percentage of cases (39%).

Severe hypertension (blood pressure >160/110) was noted during pregnancy in 30% of cases and persisted after pregnancy in 4%.

While Kitzmiller et al (1981) stated that 'the expected rate of decline in renal function was not accelerated' by pregnancy, and this is the view expressed in the recent review from the same group (Coombs & Kitzmiller 1991), they did not present data on the rate of decline of renal function before, during and after pregnancy.

They did not observe the anticipated increase in creatinine clearance during pregnancy (Fig. 6.9–2) and the creatinine clearance was lower and serum creatinine levels higher after pregnancy.

The data presented by Reece et al (1990) detailing the rate of decline of renal function before, during and after pregnancy suggest that pregnancy has no adverse effect on renal function in women with diabetic nephropathy. These authors studied renal function before, during and after pregnancy in 11 women. Their data are summarized in Figure 6.9–3. There is no significant difference between the slope of the line representing the reciprocal of the creatinine clearance in these 11 pregnancies before, during or

Table 6.9.1   Maternal complications (from Kitzmiller et al 1978)

No.	Class	Pregnancy headache	Keto-acidosis	Pyelo-nephritis	General oedema	Polyhy-dramnios	Premature labour	Pre-eclampsia	Transient hyper-tension	Chronic hyper-tension	Thyroid disease
13	A									1	
30	B	2	1		2	8	3	1			3
57	C		2	1	4	19	3	3	4		6
37	D	1	1	1	2	15	2	3	1	2	
8	F				5	4	1			4	
2	R					1					
147		3 (2%)	4 (3%)	13 (1%)	47 (9%)	9 (31%)	7 (6%)	6 (5%)	7 (4%)	9 (5%)	(6%)

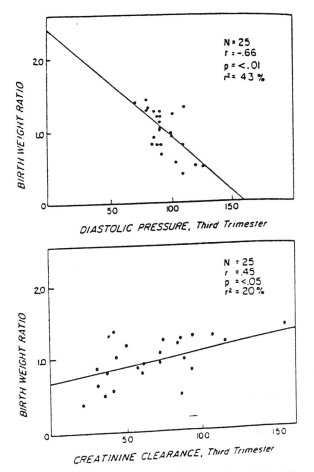

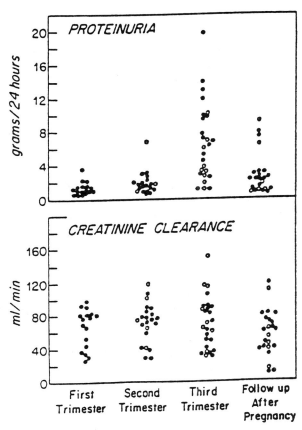

Fig. 6.9–1 Relationship between birth weight and diastolic blood pressure and creatinine clearance. (From Kitzmiller et al 1981, with permission.)

Fig. 6.9–2 Urine protein levels and creatinine clearance during pregnancy in women with diabetes in Kitzmiller's study. (From Kitzmiller et al 1981, with permission.)

after pregnancy. This is in spite of the fact that 80% of the women became nephrotic during pregnancy and in spite of hypertension in all patients.

The pioneer observations of Mogensen's group (1976), subsequently confirmed by many other groups, leaves no doubt that the degree of proteinuria and the height of the blood pressure closely correlates with the rate of decline of renal function in diabetic nephropathy. While this is true of almost all forms of renal disease it is best documented in diabetic nephropathy. Figure 6.9–2 illustrates quite clearly that several of the patients in Kitzmiller et al's (1981) study had much more protein in the urine after the pregnancy than was present in the first trimester. This

implies that they had a worse prognosis attributable to their degree of proteinuria after the pregnancy than at the beginning of pregnancy. It is reasonable to attribute this rise in protein to the pregnancy because the documented increase in proteinuria occurred during pregnancy.

It may thus be argued that pregnancy in patients with diabetic nephropathy may affect their prognosis because it is associated with a permanent increase in proteinuria. Likewise, severe hypertension with levels above 168/110 mmHg observed in 30% of women during pregnancy must be regarded as a bad prognostic feature even if hypertension of this marked degree persisted after pregnancy in only 4% of cases.

Transient nephrotic syndrome during pregnancy in women with diabetes has also been documented by Biesenbach & Zazgornik (1989),

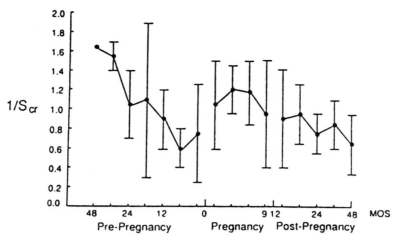

Fig. 6.9–3 Reciprocal of creatinine plotted against time in 11 women with diabetes reported by Kitzmiller et al. (From Reece et al 1990, with permission.)

who noted that this occurs in women with previous microalbuminuria but not in those with normoalbuminuria.

Severe transient nephrotic syndrome accompanied by declining renal function has also been reported (Paterson et al 1985, Weinstock et al 1988). In Weinstock's case severe nephrotic syndrome occurred in the first trimester accompanied by malignant hypertension and microangiopathic haemolytic anaemia and severe deterioration of renal function. Biopsy showed diabetic glomerulosclerosis with superimposed fibrin thrombi. Renal function remained abnormal for 3 months after the pregnancy. This case resembles those described in patients with membranoproliferative glomerulonephritis (see 6.6.5) except for a more serious maternal outcome in the latter cases.

The increase in proteinuria and the hypertension which commonly develops in pregnancy in women with diabetic nephropathy make it possible that in the long term these women may progress more rapidly to renal failure as a result of pregnancy. Individual cases such as the one described by Weinstock et al (1988) undoubtedly deteriorated as a result of the pregnancy. Biesenback et al (1992) have recently reported on pregnancy in 5 diabetic patients with impaired renal function (creatinine clearance <80 ml/min). The rate of decline of renal function was more rapid during pregnancy.

REFERENCES

Biesenbach G, Zazgornik J 1989 Incidence of transient nephrotic syndrome during pregnancy in diabetic women with and without pre-existing microalbuminuria. British Medical Journal 299: 366–367
Biesenbach G, Stöger H, Zazgornik J 1992 Influence of pregnancy on progression of diabetic nephropathy and subsequent requirement of renal replacement therapy. Nephrology, Dialysis, Transplantation 7: 105–109
Biesenbach et al (1992) have recently reported on pregnancy in 5 diabetic patients with impaired renal function (Creatinine clearance <80 ml/min). The rate of decline of renal function was more rapid during pregnancy.
Coombs C A, Kitzmiller J L 1991 Diabetic nephropathy and pregnancy. Clinical Obstetrics and Gynecology 34: 505–515
Hayslett J P, Reece E A 1987a Managing diabetic patients with nephropathy and other vascular complications. Baillières Clinical Obstetrics and Gynecology 1: 939–955
Hayslett J P, Reece E A 1987b Effect of diabetic nephropathy in pregnancy. American Journal of Kidney Diseases 9: 344–349
Kitzmiller J L, Cloherty J P, Younger M D et al 1978 Diabetic pregnancy and perinatal morbidity. American Journal of Obstetrics and Gynecology 131: 560–580
Kitzmiller J L, Brown E R, Phillippe M et al 1981 Diabetic nephropathy and perinatal outcome. American Journal of Obstetrics and Gynecology 141: 741–751
Mogensen C E 1976 Progression of nephropathy in long-term diabetics with proteinuria and effect of initial anti-hypertensive treatment. Scandinavian Journal of Clinical and Laboratory Investigation 36: 383
Oppe T E, Hsia D Y, Gillis S S 1957 Pregnancy and the diabetic mother. Lancet 1: 353
Paterson K, Lunan C B, MacCuish A C 1985 Severe transient nephrotic syndrome in diabetic pregnancy. British Medical Journal 291: 1612
Pedersen J, Pedersen L M 1965 Prognosis of the outcome of

pregnancies in diabetics. A new classification. Acta Endocrinologica 50: 70

Reece A E, Coustan D R, Hayslett J P et al 1988 Diabetic nephropathy: pregnancy performance and fetal/maternal outcome. American Journal of Obstetrics and Gynecology 159: 56–66

Reece E A, Winn H N, Hayslett J P et al 1990 Does pregnancy alter the rate of progression of diabetic nephropathy? American Journal of Perinatology 7: 193–197

Simms E A H, Krantz K E 1958 Serial studies of renal function during pregnancy and the puerperium in normal women. Journal of Clinical Investigation 37: 1764–1774

Weinstock R S, Kopecky R T, Jones D B et al 1988 Rapid development of nephrotic syndrome, hypertension, and haemolytic anaemia early in pregnancy in patients with IDDM. Diabetes Care 11: 416–421

White P 1965 Pregnancy and diabetes medical aspects. Medical Clinics of North America 49: 1015

6.10 MISCELLANEOUS RENAL DISEASES AND PREGNANCY.

6.10.1 Polycystic disease of the kidney

Considering the fact that polycystic disease of the kidney is a relatively common condition, it is surprising how little has been written about experience with pregnancy and polycystic renal disease.

Polycystic disease is the cause of end stage renal failure in 5–10% of patients reaching end stage renal failure. Renal failure commonly develops over the age of 40 so that few women would present in pregnancy with impaired renal function due to this cause.

One of the largest studies was carried out by Milutinovic et al (1983) who compared the results in pregnancy of 76 women with polycystic disease and 61 women with a family history of polycystic disease but normal kidneys. The women with polycystic kidneys were as fertile as those with normal kidneys. It is not surprising that women with cystic kidneys were more likely to develop hypertension and other complications in pregnancy (37% compared with 13%). Of women with polycystic disease 32% had hypertension prior to pregnancy compared with 6% of the women with no renal cysts; 20% of women with polycystic disease were hypertensive in the first trimester. Superimposed preeclampsia was rare, occurring in only 3% of women with cystic kidneys and in none of the control group. Increased numbers of pregnancies in women with polycystic disease did not appear to be associated with a higher incidence

of renal failure. The study group was detected by screening relatives of patients with polycystic disease and therefore probably had good renal function at the time of the pregnancy, although this is not stated.

A recent study has been reported by Jungers and colleagues from Paris. The fetal loss rate was 23%, including patients who had first trimester abortions. Unfortunately, in analysing the effects of renal failure and hypertension, Jungers combined patients with polycystic disease and reflux nephropathy. He found that in patients with these two diseases impaired renal function and hypertension influenced the rate of fetal loss. At follow up he found a much higher percentage of patients with chronic renal failure (44%) and permanent hypertension (86%) in those with polycystic disease than in those with reflux nephropathy.

Polycystic disease of the kidney usually runs a slowly progressive course and hence we attributed the rapid decline in renal function during pregnancy in a patient with impaired renal function, whose course we reported, to be the effect of the pregnancy (Kincaid-Smith et al 1967).

Two other patients with polycystic disease and impaired renal function reported by Katz et al (1979, 1980) did not show significant deterioration during pregnancy.

6.10.2 Pregnancy and renal tumours

Because renal carcinoma is rare in women under 50 years of age, it is of interest that so many cases of renal carcinoma in pregnancy have been recorded. Walker & Knight (1986) reported 2 new cases and reviewed the literature and found 35 cases of renal cell carcinoma; Table 6.10.2–1, which is reproduced from their report, details all the primary renal neoplasms reported prior to 1986.

The presenting features classical for renal carcinoma — namely, the triad of haematuria, loin pain and a palpable mass — were the same in patients presenting in pregnancy. The majority of cases in pregnancy were diagnosed because of the presence of a renal mass (88%).

Loin pain was the second most frequent presenting symptom seen in 50% of cases and all

Table 6.10.2–1   Primary renal neoplasms in pregnancy
(from Walker & Knight, 1986)

Type of tumour	No.	%
Renal cell carcinoma	35	50
Angiomyolipoma	16	23
Nephrostomata	5	7
Adenomas	3	4
Haemangiomyxoadenosarcoma	1	1.4
Carcinoidal	1	1.4
Angiosarcoma	1	1.4
Juxtaglomerular cell tumour	1	1.4
Papillary fibroma of the renal pelvis	1	1.4
Osteoadenopapilloma destruens of the renal capsule	1	1.4
Adenocarcinoma of the renal pelvis	1	1.4
Unclassified	4	6
Total	70	100

but 1 of these also had a palpable mass. Macroscopic haematuria was seen less frequently as a presenting symptom during pregnancy than is usual in other patients with renal cell carcinoma. The complete triad was seen in 26% of cases.

Of pregnant patients with tumours 18% were hypertensive and 21% had fever — one of the paraneoplastic features of renal cell carcinoma. Only 9% of women suffered weight loss.

The recommended treatment of renal cell carcinoma in pregnancy is radical excision as soon as the diagnosis is made. The outlook remains poor.

Angiomyolipoma is the second most frequent neoplasm (Table 6.10.2–1); such tumours may be associated with tuberous sclerosis. Some 80% of patients with tuberous sclerosis have angiomyolipomas and they are usually bilateral and multiple (Lipman et al 1987). Although these tumours are benign, a high percentage of cases diagnosed in pregnancy is associated with massive haemorrhage.

Pregnancy outcome in survivors of Wilms' tumour in childhood has been studied by Li et al (1987). Those who were irradiated in childhood had an adverse outcome in 30% of cases. There were 17 perinatal deaths and 17 other low birth weight infants in the 34 adverse outcomes. This represents an increased perinatal mortality rate with a relative risk of 7.9 compared with Caucasians in the United States. In contrast, an adverse outcome of pregnancy was not recorded in any one of 13 pregnancies in women who had not been irradiated.

All these women had one kidney but details on renal function and hypertension in mothers were not available.

REFERENCES

Jungers P, Forget D, Henry-Amer M, Albouze G, Fournier P, Vischer U, Droz D, Noël L-M, Grunfeld P-P 1986 Chronic kidney disease and pregnancy. In: Grunfeld J P, Maxwell M H, Bach J F, Crosnier J, Funck-Brentans (eds) Advancer in nephrology 15: 103–141
Katz M, Quagliorello J, Young B K 1979 Severe polycystic kidney disease in pregnancy. Obstetrics and Gynecology 53: 119–123
Katz A I, Davison J M, Hayslett J P et al 1980 Pregnancy in women with kidney disease. Kidney International 18: 192–206
Kincaid-Smith P, Fairley K F, Bullen M 1967 Kidney disease and pregnancy. Medical Journal of Australia 2: 1155–1159
Li F P, Gimbrere K, Gelber R D et al 1987 Outcome of pregnancy in survivors of Wilms' Tumor. Journal of the American Medical Association 257: 216–210
Lipman J C, Loughlin K, Tumeh S S 1987 Bilateral renal masses in a pregnant patient with tuberous sclerosis. Investigative Radiology 22: 912–915
Milutinovic J, Fialkow P J, Agodoa L Y et al 1983 Fertility and pregnancy complications in women with autosomal dominant polycystic kidney disease. Obstetrics and Gynecology 61: 566–570
Walker J L, Knight E L 1986 Renal cell carcinoma in pregnancy. Cancer 58: 2343–2347

6.11   PREGNANCY IN WOMEN WITH SEVERELY IMPAIRED RENAL FUNCTION AND WOMEN ON DIALYSIS

In 1971 Goldsmith et al reported on the use of haemodialysis for the treatment of fulminating preeclampsia at 28 weeks. In spite of apparent success in the latter case there has been little enthusiasm for the use of haemodialysis for the treatment of preeclampsia. In retrospect it may have been the heparinization over the whole period of haemodialysis which improved the manifestations of preeclampsia as reported by Whitworth & Fairley (1973). In the same year Confortini et al (1971) reported a full term successful pregnancy in a patient on maintenance haemodialysis.

A further way in which dialysis has been used in pregnancy is in the early dialysis of women who have severely impaired renal function but in whom dialysis is not yet warranted for any reason other than the pregnancy (Cohen et al 1988).

In the 2 cases reported by the above authors the pregnancy adversely affected the renal function, the serum creatinine rising from 2.5 mg/100 ml to 4.7 mg/100 ml in 1 patient who had glomerulonephritis and from 4.5 mg/100 ml to 12.1 mg/100 ml in a patient with reflux nephropathy. The authors concluded that dialysis contributed to the successful outcome of pregnancy and that because the patients were in advanced renal failure the impact of the pregnancy on the progression of their renal failure was of little relevance.

In 1967 we reported the results of 11 pregnancies in 9 patients with impaired renal function (blood urea above 50 mg/100 ml in early pregnancy). Although these 11 pregnancies resulted in live babies in 9 cases, serious deterioration in renal function occurred in 5 of the 9 women resulting in death or end stage renal failure. After many years of controversy surrounding our early report it is now accepted that if the serum creatinine is over 1.5–2.0 mg/ 100 ml (a similar level to a blood urea of 50 mg% during pregnancy) the likelihood of deterioration in renal function during pregnancy is high (Hou et al 1985, Surian et al 1984, Becker et al 1985, 1986).

Because a patient with a serum creatinine of 1.5–2.0 mg/100 ml can live for many years in a stable condition before developing end stage renal failure, we remain conservative in counselling such patients about pregnancy because pregnancy is likely to have an adverse effect on the course of their renal disease.

Where patients with a raised serum creatinine are keen to undertake pregnancy we have found that treatment using plasma exchange rather than dialysis may preserve renal function while achieving a successful pregnancy (d'Apice et al 1980). Figures 6.5.1–1 and 6.5.1–2 illustrate the course in pregnancy in a patient with severely impaired renal function due to reflux nephropathy.

In reflux nephropathy, pregnancy is particularly likely to cause deterioration in renal function if the serum creatinine is above 2 mg/100 ml (Becker et al 1986). In contrast women with reflux nephropathy who do not become pregnant but have a serum creatinine of 2 mg/100 ml may have stable renal function for a decade or more.

The patients illustrated in Figures 6.5.1–1 and 6.5.1–2 showed stable renal function during and after pregnancy. Pregnancy was successful and the fact that renal function did not deteriorate may well have been due to the plasma exchange treatment because no other reports have described stable renal function during and after pregnancy in patients with reflux nephropathy with this degree of renal functional impairment. We have studied 2 such patients in whom function remained stable.

We believe that plasma exchange is of value in such patients because it reduces the fibrinogen level. Fibrin deposition in the kidney is a manifestation of preeclampsia and seems to play an important role in the deterioration in renal function which occurs during pregnancy in patients with impaired renal function (Kincaid-Smith & Fairley 1987).

6.11.1 Pregnancy in women on maintenance dialysis

Since Confortini et al's report in 1971, successful pregnancy has been reported in many women on dialysis. Both haemodialysis and peritoneal dialysis have been used (Hou 1987, Redrow et al 1988).

The European Dialysis and Transplant Association reported 115 pregnancies among 13 000 women of child bearing age on dialysis, so that the incidence of pregnancy is low. In 1986 Challah et al reported 35 successful pregnancies in women on dialysis but 15 had become pregnant prior to commencing dialysis and the likelihood of successful pregnancy while on maintenance dialysis is probably below 20%.

Maternal complications are frequent in women requiring dialysis during pregnancy. If women are started on dialysis because they are pregnant, at a time before dialysis would normally be started for renal indications, they usually require continuing maintenance dialysis after the pregnancy.

Hypertension is a frequent complication in pregnant women on dialysis and severe hypertension (diastolic blood pressure above 110 mmHg) was recorded in 9 of 32 patients reviewed by Hou (1987).

Table 6.11.1–1   Cause for premature delivery (from Hou 1987, with permission)

Cause	No.	%
Premature labour	9	45
Fetal distress	3	15
Ruptured membranes	1	5
Hypertension	2	10
Haemorrhage	4	29
Intrauterine growth retardation	1	5

The blood pressure usually responds to conventional antihypertensive medication.

Anaemia is also common and a third of patients require transfusions during pregnancy (Hou et al 1987). The fetal outcome is poor, many pregnancies ending in spontaneous fetal loss. Although it is difficult to give an accurate figure for foetal loss, it is probably underestimated, particularly early fetal loss.

Premature delivery is the rule rather than the exception in women on dialysis; 20 of 29 infants reviewed by Hou (1987) were delivered before 36 weeks of gestation. Table 6.11.1–1 gives the causes for premature delivery in these cases.

The fetal weights in 30 infants reviewed by Hou (1987) showed that 8 of the infants were below the tenth percentile, 5 of them in association with severe maternal hypertension. Brem et al (1988), however, recently reported 3 live births in which there was no evidence of intrauterine growth retardation, the infants being the appropriate size for their gestational age.

Redrow et al (1988) in data from a survey of American nephrologists, reported on 8 pregnancies in 7 women on peritoneal dialysis and 6 pregnancies in women on haemodialysis. The results in these patients were good although the patients were selected; 10 of 15 pregnancies were successful, including 5 of 8 patients on peritoneal dialysis.

These authors confirmed the high rate of fetal and maternal complications in pregnancies undertaken by patients who require dialysis. They concluded that continuous ambulatory peritoneal dialysis offers several advantages: the biochemical environment is more constant on peritoneal dialysis, the haematocrit level is higher and there are fewer episodes of hypotension. The intraperitoneal route of administration is an advantage for insulin in diabetic patients and magnesium in premature labour.

REFERENCES

Becker G, Fairley K F, Whitworth J A 1985 Pregnancy exacerbates glomerular disease. American Journal of Kidney Diseases 4: 266–272

Becker G B, Ihle B U, Fairley K F et al 986 Effect of pregnancy on moderate renal failure in reflux nephropathy. British Medical Journal 292: 796

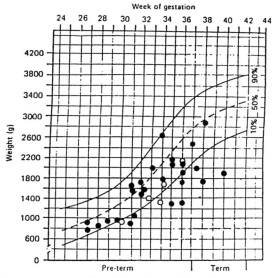

Fig. 6.11.1–1   Fetal weights in 30 infants review by Hou. (From Hou 1987, with permission.)

Brem A S, Singer D, Anderson L et al 1988 Infants of azotemic mothers: a report of three live births. American Journal of Kidney Diseases 12: 299–303

Challah S, Wing A, Broyer M et al 1986 Successful pregnancy in women on regular dialysis treatment and women with a functioning transplant In: Andreucci V F (ed) The kidney in pregnancy. Martinus Nijhoff, Boston, p 185–194

Cohen D, Frenkel Y, Maschiach S et al 1988 Dialysis during pregnancy in advanced chronic renal failure patients: outcome and progression. Clinical Nephrology 29: 144–148

Confortini P, Galanti G, Ancona G et al 1971 Full term pregnancy and successful delivery in a patient on chronic haemodialysis. Proceedings of the European Dialysis and Transplant Association 8: 74–80

d'Apice A J F, Reti L L, Pepperill R J et al 1980 Treatment of severe preeclampsia by plasma exchange. Australian and New Zealand Journal of Obstetrics and Gynaecology 20: 231–235

Goldsmith H J, Menzies D N, De Boer C H et al 1971 Delivery of healthy infant after five weeks' dialysis treatment for fulminating toxaemia of pregnancy. Lancet 2: 738–741

Hou S 1987 Peritoneal dialysis and haemodialysis in pregnancy. Bailliére's Clinical Obstetrics and Gynaecology 1: 1009–1025

Hou S, Grossman S, Madias N 1985 Pregnancy in women with renal disease and moderate renal insufficiency. American Journal of Medicine. 78: 185–194

Kincaid-Smith P, Fairley K F 1987 Renal disease in pregnancy. Three controversial areas: mesangial IgA nephropathy, focal glomerular sclerosis (focal and segmental hyalinosis and sclerosis), and reflux nephropathy. American Journal of Kidney Diseases 9: 328–333

Redrow M, Cherem L, Elliott J, et al 1988 Dialysis in the management of pregnancy patients with renal insufficiency. Medicine 67: 199–208

Surian M, Imbasciati E, Cosci P et al 1984 Glomerular disease and pregnancy. Nephron 36: 101–105

Whitworth J A, Fairley K F 1973 Heparin in the treatment of preeclamptic toxaemia. In: P Kincaid-Smith, T H Mathew, E L Becker (eds) Glomerulonephritis: morphology, natural history and treatment (Part 2). Wiley, New York, p 1027–1029

6.12 PREGNANCY AND RENAL TRANSPLANTATION

6.12.1 Pregnancy after renal transplantation

The first successful pregnancy in a patient who had received a renal transplant was recorded by Murray et al (1963) in a patient who had received a kidney from her identical twin sister.

The results of pregnancy in women with renal allografts have been the subject of many reviews (Rifle & Traeger 1975, Fine 1982, Davison & Lindheimer 1984, Penn et al 1986, Davison 1987a,b). In the latter publication 2000 pregnancies were reviewed.

The time after transplantation varies from 4 weeks to 13 years (average 40 months). The results appear to be better 2–5 years after transplantation (Davison & Lindheimer 1982). In most series, the majority of patients have received cadaveric grafts.

The success rate for pregnancy after renal transplantation is much higher than that in women on dialysis. If pregnancies progress beyond the first trimester, 90% are successful.

Spontaneous (16%) and therapeutic (22) abortions are common in most series. Ectopic pregnancy has been reported and may be more frequent in renal transplant recipients than in normal pregnancies (Scott 1978).

The overall rate of complications in pregnancy is high, particularly in women who develop complications prior to 28 weeks' gestation (Table 6.12.1–1)

If the function of the transplant kidney is impaired above a serum creatinine of 0.18 mmol/l, deterioration in renal function frequently occurs and persists after delivery in some 15% of all patients (Davison 1987b).

Women who have received renal transplants are likely to be on one or more immunosuppressive drugs at the time of conception. The most frequent drugs taken by renal allograft recipients during pregnancy are azathioprine steroids and cyclosporin A. All these drugs have potential adverse effects on the fetus and the consequences for the pregnancy may be serious.

Table 6.12.1–1 Pregnancy in renal allograft recipients: prospects (from Davison 1987a, with permission)

Problems in pregnancy (%)	Successful obstetric outcome (%)	Problems in long-term (%)
46	92 (73)	11 (24)

Estimates based on 819 women in 1025 pregnancies which attained at least 28 weeks' gestation (1961–1987). Figures in parentheses refer to prospects when complications developed prior to 28 weeks.

Table 6.12.1–2   Possible effects of immunosuppression during pregnancy (from Davison 1987, derived from data of Pirson et al 1985, with permission)

	No. of women	Pregnancies	Oligohydramnios (%)	Intrauterine growth retardation (%)	Meconium (%)	Fetal distress in labour (%)
Renal transplants	18	20	20	40	45	25
Controls	3410	5000	2	8	11	2

Table 6.12.1–2 records some of the possible effects of immunosuppression during pregnancy in a series of 20 pregnancies.

Because of the high incidence of intrauterine growth retardation, the average birth weights are low in women with renal transplants, and preterm delivery is the rule (45–60%) rather than the exception.

In addition to the contribution of immunosuppressive drugs and impaired renal function, it has been suggested that congenital cytomegalovirus infection may contribute to fetal growth retardation (Evans et al 1975.

Neonatal complications include respiratory distress syndrome, leucopenia, thrombocytopenia, adrenocortical insufficiency and infection (Fine 1982).

Maternal deaths have been recorded in 8% of women who undertook pregnancy, 8–82 months after pregnancy The maternal death rate is therefore high compared with that in normal women. Rifle & Treager (1975) reported one death from

infection following rupture of the uterus, clearly attributable to pregnancy; Table 6.12.1–3 summarizes the other maternal deaths which occurred during pregnancy or in the post-partum period.

Another important aspect of pregnancy in renal transplant recipients is the effect of the pregnancy on renal function and graft loss; Hou (1989) has recently summarized the published data on this and Table 6.12.1–3 is derived from her review.

When renal function declines in pregnancy or graft loss occurs, it may be difficult to determine whether this is due to pregnancy or represents the 'natural history' of decline in renal function in the transplanted kidney. If pregnancy is undertaken 5 or more years after transplantation, 75% of women will have worse renal function after the pregnancy than that recorded before pregnancy (Gaudier et al 1988).

Women with impaired graft function are more likely to show significant deterioration during

Table 6.12.1–3   Frequency of maternal complications of pregnancy in transplant recipients — data from six studies (from Hou 1989, with permission)

Study	Pregnancy patients	Caesarean section	Maternal death †	Decreased GFR	Graft (loss) +	Increased blood pressure ¶
Rifle & Troeger* 1975	120/103	2	3/47	(0)	11/40	22/42
Rudolph et al* 1979	440/406	1	25	(15)	132	
Penn et al 1980	56/37	0	4	(3)//	18	9/45
Whetham et al 1983	7/5	0	3/6	(2)	3	6/6
O'Donnell et al 1985	38/21	0	5	(2)	8/30	
Marushak et al 1986	24/20	0	2	(0)	6	18/24

* Denotes a study done by questionnaire. Complete data were not available for all patients and pregnancies. When incomplete data are available, the numerator is the number of patients affected and the denominator is the number of patients for whom we have information. There is some overlap between the Rudolph and Penn studies.
† Refers to maternal death during pregnancy in the immediate postpartum period, or as a result of pregnancy,.
+ The number in parentheses indicates those with decreased GFR in pregnancy who progressed to lose their grafts.
¶ When specific blood pressures are given in the study, all patients with a systolic blood pressure greater than 140 mmHg or a diastolic greater than 90 mmHg are considered hypertensive.
// Two of the women who lost their grafts stopped taking immunosuppressive medication.
GFR, glomerular filtration rate.

pregnancy and it is accepted that this is due to the pregnancy. Davison (1987a) reported that in 15 women with a serum creatinine above 0.18 mmol/l deterioration in renal function was frequent, and in 15% it persisted after delivery.

More controversy exists, however, about the likelihood of pregnancy causing deterioration in renal function in renal transplant recipients with normal renal function. Whetham et al (1983) compared two groups of women with renal transplants: one group of 5 women with 7 pregnancies and a control group of 10 women who did not become pregnant. Two women in the control group lost their grafts and 2 of 5 women who became pregnant lost their grafts 7 and 18 months after pregnancy. Both had raised serum creatinine levels before pregnancy.

A much larger review reported 25 severe rejection episodes in 400 pregnancies (Rudolph et al 1979). Among 21 where the outcome was known, 15 rejection episodes were irreversible and 6 of these patients died. In some cases rejection occurred during pregnancy in patients with previously stable renal function who had not had previous rejection episodes or had had them only in the early posttransplant period.

We have had similar experience when a woman with stable renal function a year or more after transplantation develops severe vascular rejection during pregnancy; this is quite different from the expected natural course in that patient. Furthermore, the rejection episodes during pregnancy or in the early postpartum period may be accompanied by florid vascular changes accompanied by fibrin and foam cells in vessels — a change which we have only observed in hyperacute rejection in the early postgraft period with the exception of these biopsies during pregnancy. From this we conclude that pregnancy may cause severe acute rejection in women who would not otherwise have lost their kidneys. As indicated above in Rudolph's series, loss of allograft function may lead to death of the mother. This occurred in 6 of 15 patients in his review.

Hypertension is common in renal transplant recipients and severe hypertension is also frequently observed. The drugs used to control hypertension during pregnancy in transplant patients are the same as those recommended in other forms of hypertension in pregnancy.

Proteinuria usually increases during pregnancy (Fig. 6.12–1). Based on the presence or development or increase in hypertension and proteinuria, preeclampsia is diagnosed in about 1 in 3 cases, but eclampsia is rare (Williams & Jelen 1979).

Because the lesions of acute rejection and more of preeclampsia are essentially thrombotic in nature (Kincaid-Smith 1975) we have used heparin with dipyridamole and plasma exchange in an attempt to improve the outcome of pregnancy in patients with renal allograft and impaired renal failure with some apparent success (d'Apice et al 1980).

Postpartum renal failure accompanied by oliguria and thrombotic microangiopathy has been recorded following renal transplantation (Lederer et al 1989).

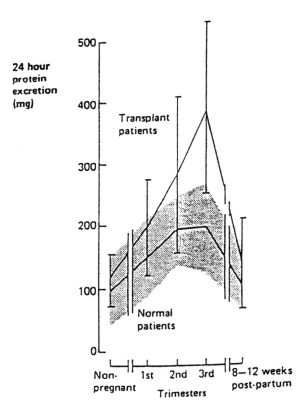

Fig. 6.12–1 Protein excretion before, during and after pregnancy in renal transplant patients. (From Davison 1987a, with permission.)

6.12.2 The impact of donor nephrectomy on pregnancy

This subject was reviewed by Buszta et al (1985) who considered the experience at the Cleveland Clinic where 23% of 191 female kidney donors had had pregnancies following donor nephrectomy for living donor transplantation; 32 of 39 pregnancies were successful 2 weeks to 9 years following donor nephrectomy. Evaluation was carried out at that time and included history examination, renal function tests and urinalysis. The results were compared with those obtained prior to donor nephrectomy.

The details of this analysis by Buszta et al (1985) are shown in Tables 6.12.2–1 and 6.12.2–2.

The serum creatinine had increased by 17% over a mean period of 7.9 years and the glomerular filtration rate (iothalamate clearance) had fallen by 24%.

The protein excretion and blood pressure were normal in each individual patient. The authors concluded that pregnancy had little impact on the woman who had undergone donor nephrectomy for living donor renal transplantation.

REFERENCES

Buszta C, Steinmuller D R, Novick A C et al 1985 Pregnancy after donor nephrectomy. Transplantation 40: 651–654
d'Apice A J F, Reti L L, Pepperell R J et al 1980 Treatment of severe preeclampsia by plasma exchange. Australian and New Zealand Journal of Obstetrics and Gynaecology 20: 231–235
Davison J M 1987a Pregnancy in renal allograft recipients: prognosis and management. Baillières Clinical Obstetrics and Gynaecology 11: 1027–1045

Table 6.12.2–1 Reevaluation post nephrectomy and pregnancy (from Buszta et al 1985, with permission)

Patient	Serum creatinine (mg/100 ml)	GFR (ml/min/1.73^2)	Urinary protein (g/24 h)	Blood pressure (mmHg)
1	1.0	90	0.08	130/80
2	1.1	77	0.05	118/70
3	1.0	71	0.05	135/85
4	1.0	93	0.03	108/70
5	1.0	81	0.08	118/72
6	1.1	85	0.01	130/70
7	1.5	76	0.02	100/50
8	1.1	84	0.09	120/70
9	1.2	75	0.04	130/70
10	1.0	81	0.07	124/82
11	1.0	100	0.04	90/68
12	1.1	82	0.09	108/78
13	1.2	78	0.04	120/80
Mean	1.10	82.5	0.05	117/72
SD	0.14	7.68	0.026	126/85

GFR, glomerular filtration rate.

Table 6.12.2–2 Glomerular filtration rate (GFR): effects of organ donation and pregnancy (from Buszta et al 1985, with permission)

Pre transplant	At reevaluation	Percentage change	Mean length of follow up (years)
Serum creatinine (mg/100 ml) 0.94 (±0.14)* (n = 13)	1.1 (± 0.14) (n = 13)	+17	7.9
GFR (ml/min/1.7 m^2) 109 (±28) (n = 8)	83 (±9) (n = 8)	−24	6.1

*SD in parentheses.

Davison J M 1987b Renal transplantation and pregnancy. American Journal of Kidney Diseases 9: 374–380

Davison J M, Lindheimer M D 1982 Pregnancy in renal transplant recipients. Journal of Reproductive Medicine 27: 613–620

Davison J M, Lindheimer M D 1984 Pregnancy in women with renal allografts. Seminars in Nephrology 4: 240–251

Evans T J, McCollum J P K, Valdimarsson H 1975 Congenital cytomegalovirus infection after maternal renal transplantation. Lancet 1: 1359–1360

Fine R N 1982 Pregnancy in renal allograft recipients. American Journal of Nephrology 2: 117–122

Gaudier F L, Santiago-Delpin E, Rivera J et al 1988 Pregnancy after renal transplantation. Surgery, Gynecology and Obstetrics 167: 533–543

Hou S 1989 Pregnancy in organ transplant recipients. Medical Clinics of North America 73: 667–683

Kincaid-Smith P 1975 Participation of intravascular coagulation in the pathogenesis of glomerular and vascular lesions. Kidney International 7: 242–253

Lederer E L, Suki W N, Truong L D 1989 Postpartum renal failure in a renal transplant patient. Transplantation 47: 717–719

Marushak A, Weber T, Bock J 1986 Pregnancy following kidney transplantation. Acta Obstetricia et Gynecologica Scandinavica 65: 557

Murray J E, Reid D E, Harrison J H et al 1963 Successful pregnancies after human renal transplantation. New England Journal of Medicine 269: 341–343

O'Donnell D, Sevitz H, Seggie J L 1985 Pregnancy after renal transplantation. Australian and New Zealand Journal of Medicine 15: 320

Penn I 1986 Pregnancy following renal transplantation. In: V E Andreucci, (ed) The kidney in pregnancy. Martinus Nijhoff, Boston, p 195–204

Penn I, Makowski E L, Harris P 1980 Parenthood following renal transplantation. Kidney International 18: 221

Pirson Y, van Lierde M, Ghysen J et al 1985 Retardation of fetal growth in patients receiving immunosuppressive therapy. New England Journal of Medicine 313: 328

Rifle G, Traeger J 1975 Pregnancy after renal transplantation: an international survey. Transplantation Proceedings 7: 723–728

Rudolph J E, Shwihizir R T, Barius S A 1979 Pregnancy in renal transplant patients: a review. Transplantation Proceedings 7: 26–29

Scott J R, Cruickshank D P, Corry R J 1978 Ectopic pregnancy in kidney transplant patients. Obstetrics and Gynecology 51: 565–568

Whetham J C G, Gardella C, Harding M 1983 Effect of pregnancy on graft function and graft survival in renal cadaver transplant patients. American Journal of Obstetrics and Gynecology 145: 193

Williams P T, Jelen J 1979 Eclampsia in a patient who had had a renal transplant. British Medical Journal 2: 972

6.13 COUNSELLING, INVESTIGATION AND MANAGEMENT OF PATIENTS WITH RENAL DISEASE IN RELATION TO PREGNANCY

We always advise women with renal disease to come with their partners to discuss pregnancy with us before they embark on pregnancy.

When renal function is normal it is only occasionally necessary to advise against pregnancy and usually when this is done it is a question of timing the pregnancy to when optimal results are likely in relation to management of the underlying renal disease. It is inappropriate, for example, for a women with renal calculi to became pregnant when a ureteric calculus is obstructing one kidney — clearly the stone should be extracted prior to pregnancy.

If a woman has a refractory urinary infection then the source of this should be sought and treated prior to pregnancy. This could be an infected stone or a blind ureteric stump and in either case the infection can only be cured by removing the cause.

In patients with glomerular disease, nephrologists are perhaps less likely to treat the glomerular disease before advising about pregnancy because a negative attitude prevails concerning treatment of glomerulonephritis. Most would perhaps agree that an active diffuse proliferative lupus glomerulonephritis should be treated prior to pregnancy but could not necessarily treat a membranous glomerulonephritis or mesangial IgA glomerulonephritis. We would treat all these in certain circumstances and believe that this not only optimizes the chance of a successful pregnancy but also reduces the likelihood of deterioration in renal function in the mother.

In membranous glomerulonephritis we, and other groups, have shown that the presence of the nephrotic syndrome is associated with a poor pregnancy outcome (Packham et al 1987). For this reason we would advise treatment of a patient with heavy proteinuria due to membranous glomerulonephritis prior to pregnancy. We find that a combination of cyclophosphamide, dipyridamole and warfarin is effective in reducing proteinuria in most patients, as demonstrated in the Australian controlled trial of this combination (Fig. 6.13–1).

This treatment often reverses the membranous lesion as well as reducing proteinuria (Kincaid-Smith 1975). We have supervised up to 3 successful and uneventful pregnancies in individual patients with treated membranous glomerulo-

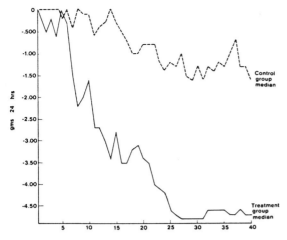

Fig. 6.13–1   Significant reduction in urine protein level in membranous glomerulonephritis in the threated group in a randomized prospective trial of cyclophosphamide, warfarin and dipyridamole.

nephritis, whereas others have recorded malignant hypertension and deterioration in renal function in women with membranous glomerulonephritis and the nephrotic syndrome (Studd & Blainey 1969).

Mesangial IgA glomerulonephritis has a variable outcome in pregnancy but in active cases crescents may develop and renal function may deteriorate during pregnancy (Packham et al 1988a,b, Fairley & Packham 1989).

In mesangial IgA glomerulonephritis a continuous high urinary erythrocyte count has the strongest predictive value for progression (Nicholls et al 1984) and when the count is high it reflects crescents (Bennett & Kincaid-Smith 1983).

Several treatments, including quite simple ones, have been shown in controlled trials to reduce the urinary erythrocyte count: among these are tetracycline and phenytoin as well as more aggressive treatment such as steroids and cyclophosphamide. We would treat patients using one of these methods prior to pregnancy if the urinary erythrocyte count was high.

The investigations which we would do prior to pregnancy are plasma and creatinine levels and a creatinine clearance to assess renal function. Quantitative proteinuria and a careful evaluation of urine microscopy are useful in assessing activity of the glomerular disease. Culture is obviously important where infection is a consideration.

If the urinary erythrocyte count is high as an isolated phenomenon, the patient is likely to have one of two diagnoses, namely mesangial IgA glomerulonephritis or thin basement membrane disease (Kincaid-Smith 1990), but another disease which may present as isolated microscopy haematuria is lupus glomerulonephritis. In our view a renal biopsy should be carried out prior to pregnancy, not only to determine the diagnosis but to determine the histological lesions within each diagnostic category. Lesions are likely to be mild in thin basement membrane disease and pregnancy is usually uneventful in such patients. The histological lesion affects the outcome of pregnancy in mesangial IgA glomerulonephritis (Packham et al 1988a) and quite severe lesions, including crescents, may be present.

In a patient with isolated microscopic haematuria due to lupus glomerulonephritis, we would certainly treat active lupus glomerulonephritis prior to pregnancy.

If tests prior to pregnancy showed that renal function was impaired with a serum creatinine of 0.15–0.20 mmol/l, we would warn the patient of the very well documented risk that further deterioration is likely to occur during pregnancy (Becker et al 1986, Hou et al 1985).

Women with renal disease also need to know about the significantly increased risk of fetal loss (Packham et al 1989), such that a woman may develop end stage renal failure as a result of pregnancy and not achieve the desired living baby.

6.13.1 Management during pregnancy in women with underlying renal disease

Because maternal and fetal complications are more likely in women with renal disease, close supervision in pregnancy is recommended both by the obstetrician and by the nephrologist, who should collaborate closely in the supervision of pregnancy. Careful blood pressure monitoring is essential through the whole pregnancy.

We normally see a patient with renal disease at the end of the first trimester when renal function tests are carried out to assess if the kidney has responded with the anticipated improvement in renal function. Quantitative assessment of urine protein and careful urine microscopy are valuable in assessing the activity of the renal disease at this time.

A new method of assessment which may prove of value is the uterine artery doppler waveform. We have certainly encountered very abnormal uterine artery waveforms at about 20 weeks' gestation which improve dramatically with treatment (Fig. 6.13.1–1).

If sudden deterioration occurs in any of the features which are being observed we will often carry out a renal biopsy during pregnancy (Packham & Fairley 1987).

The rate of complications is low and a biopsy may provide valuable information and influence treatment in the individual patient. We would, for example, use plasma exchange in the woman with severe diffuse proliferative lupus nephritis.

Certain clinical and laboratory observations are made at regular intervals throughout pregnancy. The more serious the renal disease the more frequent the observations. Blood pressure, weight gain, proteinuria are perhaps the most important features to follow, but in addition, urea, uric acid and creatinine are monitored monthly. Urine microscopy in skilled hands provides a sensitive index of activity of the renal disease and of the onset of preeclampsia when an increase in erythrocytes, erythrophagocytosis and casts is seen. From about 26 weeks' gestation, haemoglobin, haematocrit and platelet count are added to the list of investigations repeated on a regular basis, and selected patients may require liver function tests.

From 28 weeks of gestation most patients with renal disease need to have clinical and biochemical abnormalities monitored on a weekly basis.

When superimposed preeclampsia develops we admit the patient to hospital and carry out daily clinical monitoring and investigations.

Admission to hospital allows careful fetal monitoring by cardiotachometry. Ultrasound to document intrauterine growth retardation and amniotic fluid volume and doppler velocimetry may also be useful in late pregnancy. Amniocentesis is occasionally used.

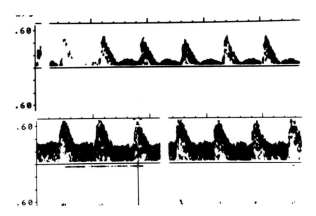

Fig. 6.13.1–1 Doppler wave form in the uterine artery in a woman with severe renal disease (focal and segmental hyalinosis and sclerosis) who developed the nephrotic syndrome and severe hypertension at 20 weeks gestation. The upper curve shows the wave form at 20 weeks gestation before plasma exchange treatment. The lower curve shows the considerably improved wave from at 22 weeks after plasma exchange therapy which was continued until delivery. All clinical features improved as did a severe active lesion on renal biopsy. The pregnancy continued to 36 weeks when a live baby was delivered.

6.13.2 Treatment which can be used early in pregnancy and may prevent superimposed preeclampsia in women with renal disease

Because the increase in vascular reactivity and increased sensitivity to angiotensin come on early in the second trimester and because the abnormalities in placental vessels characteristic of preeclampsia also come on at this time, measures arrived at preventing preeclampsia are more likely to succeed than are measures aimed at treating established preeclampsia.

Beaufils et al (1985) showed that aspirin and dipyridamole given from 12–14 weeks' gestation considerably improved the outcome of pregnancy in women with high risk pregnancy or underlying renal disease.

We have shown in a controlled trial that a combination of dipyridamole and subcutaneous low dose heparin (7500–10 000 units twice daily) given from 14–16 weeks' of gestation to the end of pregnancy reduces the risk of hypertension and proteinuria in patients with renal disease (Table

Table 6.13.2–1 Randomized controlled trial of heparin and dipyridamol from 14–16 weeks gestation in women with renal disease.

	TREATED	CONTROL
Number	10	11
Hypertension	0	6*
Proteinuria	0	5*
Deterioration in renal function	1	5

(p*<0.01)

6.13.2–1). In this series fetal loss occurred in 5/11 control patients and no treated patient.

6.13.3 Treatment after the onset of preeclampsia

The only treatment that will rapidly and predictably reverse the features of preeclampsia is delivery of the baby, and with advances in neonatal paediatrics this is the method of choice in many cases.

Bed rest may reverse some of the features of preeclampsia including hypertension, proteinuria and hyperuricaemia.

In a series of 9 patients treated with heparin in the days before neonatal care was as effective as it is at this time, treatment seemed to achieve stabilization of clinical and biochemical abnormalities and achieve more mature infants (Whitworth & Fairley 1973).

In more severe cases with earlier onset preeclampsia we have used plasma exchange in the latter weeks or months of pregnancy to achieve sufficient fetal maturity for survival (Fig 6.5.1–1).

Although there is no evidence that blood pressure control in preeclampsia does anything to reverse the disease process or to increase the fetal survival it is often necessary to avoid risks for the mother.

Methyldopa is the drug which has been most widely used in the control of hypertension in pregnancy. Other drugs which are safe and effective are β-adrenergic blocking agents, hydralazine, clonidine, labetalol and nifedipine.

If rapid lowering of the blood pressure is necessary, vasodilator such as hydralazine or nifedipine are effective. Intravenous diazoxide often used in the past is now less popular because it decreases placental blood flow.

REFERENCES

Beaufils M, Uzan S, Donsimoni R et al 1985 Prevention of preeclampsia by early anti-platelet therapy. Lancet 1: 840–842

Becker G J, Ihle B U, Fairley K F et al 1986 Effect of pregnancy on moderate renal failure in reflux nephropathy. British Medical Journal 292: 796–798

Bennet W M, Kincaid-Smith P 1982 Macroscopic haematuria in mesangial IgA nephropathy: clinical pathological correlations. Kidney International 23: 393–400

Fairley C K, Packham D K 1989 Glomerular crescents and pregnancy. American Journal of Kidney Diseases 13: 250–252

Hou S, Grossman S, Madias N 1985 Pregnancy in women with renal disease and moderate renal insufficiency. American Journal of Medicine 78: 185–194

Kincaid-Smith P (ed) 1975 The kidney — a clinicopathological study. Blackwell Scientific, Oxford, p 164

Kincaid-Smith P 1991 Unexplained haematuria. British Medical Journal 302: 177

Nicholls K M, Fairley K F Dowling J P et al 1984 The clinical course of mesangial IgA nephropathy. Quarterly Journal of Medicine 53: 227–250

Packham D K, Fairley K F 1987 Renal biopsy: indications and complications in pregnancy. British Journal of Obstetrics and Gynaecology 94: 935–939

Packham D K, North R A, Fairley K F et al 1987 Membranous glomerulonephritis and pregnancy. Clinical Nephrology 28: 56–64

Packham D K, North R A, Fairley K F, et al 1988a IgA glomerulonephritis and pregnancy. Clinical Nephrology 30: 15–21

Packham D K, Fairley K F, Whitworth J A et al 1988b Comparison of pregnancy outcome between normotensive and hypertensive women with primary glomerulonephritis. Clinical and Experimental Hypertension B6: 387–400

Packham D K, North R A, Fairley K F et al 1989 Primary glomerulonephritis and pregnancy. Quarterly Journal of Medicine 266: 537–553

Studd J W W, Blainey J D 1969 Pregnancy and the nephrotic syndrome. British Medical Journal 1: 276–280

Whitworth J A, Fairley K F 1973 Heparin in the treatment of preeclamptic toxaemia. In: P Kincaid-Smith, T H Mathew, E L Becker (eds) Glomerulonephritis. Wiley, New York, p 1027–1029

Index